You were just a child ...
LOOKING FOR LOVE

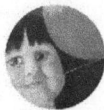

GREEN BALLOON PUBLISHING

This book is about the theoretical and practical developments of Professor Dr Franz Ruppert, known as Identity-oriented Psychotrauma Therapy (IoPT).

IoPT theory involves an in depth understanding of trauma, particularly trauma that happens very early in life, even before birth, the subsequent dynamics of this traumatisation and the potential lifelong impact.

The content of this book is oriented towards those who have some knowledge and understanding of IoPT theory and the practice method, and so a basic outline of this theory is not part of this book.

If, however, you find this book in your hands, and you do not as yet have any knowledge of IoPT theory and thinking, you might find it helpful to read another book I wrote that is a very basic introduction to this topic, entitled:

Becoming Your True Self; a Handbook for the Journey from Trauma to Healthy Autonomy. This book is currently translated into Dutch, German, Russian and Norwegian.

For further interest there are at present nine books by Professor Ruppert translated into English from their original German:

Trauma Bonding & Family Constellations

Splits in the Soul: Integrating Traumatic Experiences

Symbiosis & Autonomy: Symbiotic Trauma and Love Beyond Entanglements

Trauma Fear & Love: How the Constellation of Intention Supports Healthy Autonomy

My Body, My Trauma, My I: Setting up Intentions; Exiting my Traumabiography

Early Trauma: Pregnancy, Birth and First Years of Life

Who am I in a Traumatised and Traumatising Society

Love Lust and Trauma: The Journey towards a Healthy Sexual Identity

I want to Live, Love & Be Loved

And there are another two books of mine:

The Heart of Things: Understanding Trauma – Working with Constellations

Trauma and Identity: IoPT Theory and Practice, translated into Dutch, and shortly in German.

Most of these books have been translated into other languages. All Professor Ruppert's books were originally in German. Mine are originally in English.

www.franz-ruppert.de/

www.vivianbroughton.com

www.greenballoonbooks.co.uk

You were just a child ...
LOOKING FOR LOVE

*"Living a good life" and other IoPT essays
and thoughts*

by Vivian Broughton

"I'm the enemy of the unlived, meaningless life."
Bob Dylan ('False Prophet')

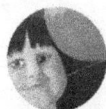

GREEN BALLOON PUBLISHING

All case studies in this book are based on real events. In order to protect
the identity of those concerned, names and, where necessary,
personal details have been altered.

Green Balloon Publishing, Steyning
www.greenballoonbooks.co.uk

ISBN 978-1-8381419-2-9

Book production by The Choir Press, Gloucester
Set in Candara

Contents

Foreword – Lucy Jameson

I first met Vivian Broughton in October 2012, when I went for an individual session with her in London, shortly followed by a group workshop. Once I had discovered IoPT, I never looked back. Ten years later, I am an IoPT facilitator myself, and I can safely say that I know myself so much better now than I did back then. I am profoundly grateful to Vivian for the part that she has played in my journey – as a practitioner, teacher, companion, colleague and friend.

It is rare that someone can be so good at what they do, and also able to write about it in such an eloquent and accessible way. Vivian's book is a joy to read: packed with useful information and reflections about the reality of trauma, coupled with a deep understanding of Franz Ruppert's theory and method, which she approaches and works with in her own unique and personal way.

I am also touched by Vivian's willingness to share her own vulnerability, through the more intimate essays that appear in these pages, and the truths that she has learned for herself about the reality of her own early experiences.

My feeling is that this book will serve as an invaluable guide for new practitioners, a useful reference point for more experienced facilitators, and a captivating read for anyone who is interested in exploring the topic of early trauma. It has touched my heart and contributed hugely to my understanding of our collective humanity.

We were all once just children, looking for love ... and we are all people for whom living a good life is a very real and joyous possibility.

Lucy Jameson,

Sussex,

August 2022

Foreword – Marta Thorsheim

Thank you, Vivian for writing this book, so full of honesty and openness, and your warm humor.

As a practitioner of some 30 years, following Franz Ruppert`s IoPT developments, and supporting as many IoPT students as I can, it is difficult to say how touched and thankful I am to him for what he has brought into the world. His way of making complex topics about trauma and human development easily available, without losing the depth and complexity, is quite extraordinary.

And then to Vivian, with all her efforts to bring even more clarity to this complexity, through her writings and her support of IoPT students.

My experience is that people, at first glance, may think IoPT is simple. However, it is only after some time that the depth and holistic nature of the theory may dawn on them. Then I find that people want to continue exploring their journey of growth, what trauma means in their life, and the effect of not having been wanted or loved. Thus, people learn more and more about themselves, and who they really are underneath the traumas they have suffered, through the theory of IoPT, and the methodology of the self-encounter, the Intention Method.

This book offers a fresh breeze, where both practitioners of IoPT, and IoPT-interested people may nod in agreement and recognition, and find new angles of understanding and insightful learning.

I especially love the way Vivian combines theory and the methodology in her writing. Every IoPT practitioner and student, and I think also IoPT-interested people, will find new insights in this book, as I did when I read it. The journey of grasping the theory of IoPT, and what it may mean for humanity in the future, takes some years. There are now an increasing number of IoPT practitioners throughout the world, and the method and theory of IoPT is being used increasingly by counsellors and coaches, thereby offering an increasing number of people a better way of living a good life.

It is easy to read an academic book about trauma and bypass our emotions, or to talk about trauma and suppress emotions. And it is just as easy to be overwhelmed by the topic of trauma and avoid it. The support of skilled IoPT practitioners may be very helpful in order to avoid falling into either of these traps.

I have travelled all over the world introducing IoPT to others, as has Vivian, and now we are experiencing people joining IoPT trainings and courses from many different countries. With this approachable book about IoPT and our search for love, Vivian has made it possible to avoid the traps along the way, and go to the core of people's issues in our search for healing from the traumas of not being wanted and loved at the beginning of our life, and then to come to love ourselves.

A heartfelt thank you to Vivian for taking the time and energy to write this book.

Marta Thorsheim

Oslo, Norway

January 2023

"Information is not necessarily the truth"

Yuval Noah Harari

"Those that fight don't listen,
and those that listen don't fight"

Fritz Perls

Introduction

This book is primarily about love; love as the basic force of life; love that is lost or never born in the relationship between mother and infant; love that is the underlying need of the child; love that is delusionary, holding us in endless hope; and love that is honest and true, based on reality, and then, possible in our relationship with ourselves, and those we truly love.

Love is the turning point from trauma to health.

Becoming 'IoPT-Informed' offers an open invitation to everyone to think about themselves from the perspective of understanding trauma, and how it has impacted them, and as an encouragement to take up the challenge to find who you really are, your true identity, and thence find love for yourself, and honest love for others.

Since one of the primary principles of IoPT[1] is the principle of autonomy and self-responsibility, this journey must be instigated and taken up by each one of us: no one can heal anyone else's trauma; we can only heal our own; no one else can do this for us. In this sense we are all individual explorers of ourselves, eventually coming to our birth right: the ability to know ourselves and live a full and satisfying and meaningful life.

Becoming 'IoPT-Informed' does indeed take us on a journey where everything can be considered through the lens of IoPT thinking, through the meaning therein. IoPT then becomes not just a theory and a therapeutic method, but a psychology and a philosophy, that can illuminate what happens in our own personal world, and in the wider political and social world. All of the major topics we are collectively struggling with every single day, and those personal musings about our own life ... all can be considered from an IoPT perspective.

As an IoPT practitioner the most important thing I have learned about the practice of IoPT is the art of saying less, speaking only if necessary and, instead, trusting the resonance process and the person exploring themselves to find the resolution. The solution is always there, in the process, not in me as the facilitator; the resonators and the enquiring

---

[1]   Identity-oriented Psychotrauma Therapy, the original theoretical developments of Professor Dr Franz Ruppert, Munich, Germany.

person together will show me what the truth is, and where the solution lies, and only then can I say something that is helpful, or perhaps I can see that my 'contribution' is not necessary at all.

These essays are, to an extent, the result of listening, and many of them come directly from a process I have facilitated or a personal process of my own. Some of the learnings stray from the actual encounter exploration itself, but raised thoughts that I pursued in my own time. Others are directly the outcome of an exploration process. Some follow the process to an extent, and others do not. Some essays are quite personal to me, and some are more general. Most of the essays are spoken to IoPT practitioners, thoughts about our work and how we think and how we practice. A few are stories I tell that illustrate something, and some are just a couple of lines, leaving the reader to think about what I have said, and fill in the gaps. On occasion an idea in one essay may reappear in another; I decided to leave them like that, because I think the idea important enough to deserve repetition in another context. In the end, all of these essays and thoughts are about love: understanding what it is, and finding it within ourselves.

As IoPT facilitators, when you start to really listen to the representatives and the enquiring person, and wait as long as you can bear to before intervening, you will learn amazing things that you have never thought of before. The IoPT process will teach you, that is the point, and if you listen you will learn. In fact, you will learn things that are not in any of the books, or perhaps they are but you may have missed them. Or perhaps you have interpreted them in a certain way, and what happens in front of you gives another angle, another truth. You will learn about yourself, and about life. Be a listening facilitator rather than a talking facilitator, that is my message.

My previous book, Trauma and Identity, aimed to be a textbook of IoPT, drawing into one place every important theoretical concept Ruppert has developed over the past 30 odd years, together with some of my own thoughts and ideas about his theories. As such, that book required careful structuring so that the topics appeared in a sequential ordering that made sense, and took the person on a reasonably logical journey through the essentials of IoPT theory and practice.

In contrast this book is a varied collection of thoughts and ideas, some full-length essays, and some short statements, all of which have IoPT thinking underlying them.

When it came to organising a structure for these essays, after some attempts to categorise, putting similar topics or types together, eventually I decided not to. In the end I liked the randomness of the topics and put these essays simply into alphabetical order according to the title. Therefore, this is not a book to be read straight through, from beginning to end. It doesn't work that way. Rather I suggest you scan the titles and see where you are drawn. The topics do not follow any sequence, and so do not need to be read in sequence. Follow your instinct and enjoy the result.

With love
Vivian Broughton
Wiltshire 2023

All references in words like 'him' or 'her' - gender references - are always referring to all unless I am talking about a specific person.

Acknowledgements

My first acknowledgement, of course, is of Professor Dr Franz Ruppert. His work over the last thirty years has provided me, and the many, many others who have decided to take themselves and their trauma seriously, with a dramatic turning point in life. I truly believe that his theoretical developments known as Identity-oriented Psychotrauma Therapy offer a profound solution to the many confusions of what it is to be human. My thanks to him.

My thanks also to Lucy Jameson who took considerable time to read the manuscript for this book and offered me many useful and constructive comments and feedback.

Thank you also to John Mitchell of Green Balloon Publishing for his extensive work in editing and preparing the final manuscript for publishing.

In addition, I thank Miles Bailey, Rachel Woodman and all at Choir Press for their support in dealing with the technology of publication.

My most profound appreciation, however, goes to all the many people who have worked with me on their own personal issues, and the increasing number of IoPT practitioners I try and support in their work. Most of the thoughts and realisations in this book have been sparked by their willingness to take themselves and their trauma seriously, and share their insights with me.

All 'intentions' in this book are real intentions set by people, however the thoughts I put to them are mine, with the aim of showing the use of IoPT theory in understanding intentions and processes. As one of my students said, my aim is to help IoPT students learn how to think when facilitating their work with clients.

Since there are no exact accounts of processes, and my inclusion of actual intentions is a device to enable me to share my thoughts from an IoPT perspective, in general I have not felt it necessary to ask permission to use the intentions. On some occasions, where I have gone further into what actually happened in the process, I have gained permission from the person whose intention I am using, but the thoughts I give about these intentions and processes are my thoughts, and may not concur with what the person gained from the process.

"The truth will set you free, but first it will piss you off."
Gloria Steinem

A Reminder

The IoPT Icon showing the splits after trauma.

Do not be misled by the simplicity of this little icon. The underlying meanings are incredibly complex and take some years to really understand.

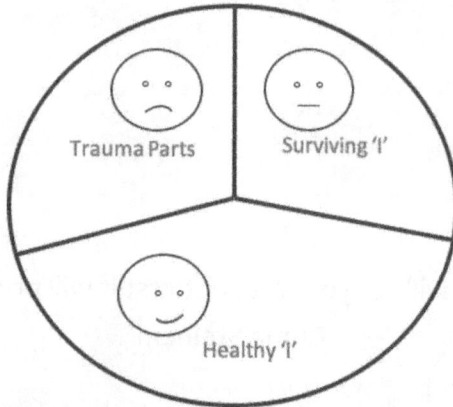

And the Traumabiography Icon. This shows the sequence of traumatisation starting at the bottom.

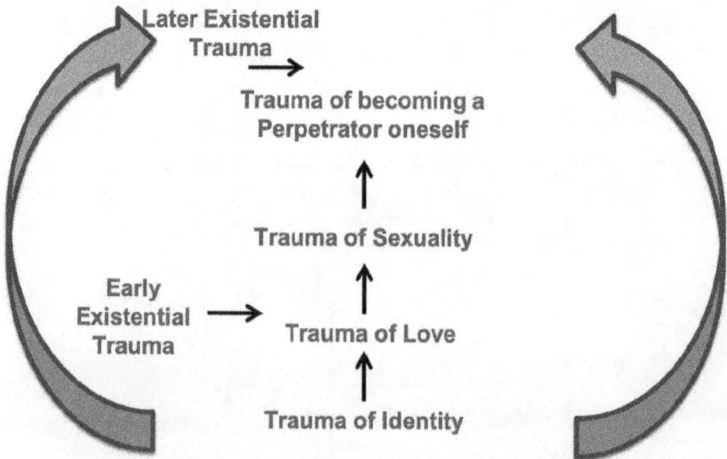

Basic Survival Strategies of these Traumas:

TRAUMA OF IDENTITY - Identification with external phenomena (the mother originally)

TRAUMA OF LOVE - Illusions of Love ("One day my mother will love me")

TRAUMA OF SEXUALITY (Not being protected) - Illusions and confusion about sexuality and safety

TRAUMA OF BECOMING A PERPETRATOR - Escalating perpetration of self and of others

The Early and Later Existential Traumas are always strongly influenced by the main Traumabiography traumas.

Abandonment ...

Intention: "I want to heal my fear of abandonment."

The word 'abandon' means a withdrawal of support.

But if we understand the Trauma of Identity, we can see that the word 'abandon' is incorrect. To abandon someone or something means there must have been a connection (support) before, that was later withdrawn, but the Trauma of Identity is the situation where there never was a connection or support right from the start. It is the trauma of not being wanted in the first place.

To hold onto the idea that your mother abandoned you, that your issue is abandonment, you hold onto the hope that there was a time before you were abandoned, and that underneath it all she loves you. But the reality in such a situation is that she didn't want you, perhaps even hated you, from the beginning.

If you keep your focus on your mother, you end up abandoning yourself.

———————⌗———————

About thinking and feeling

Thinking uses the information that comes from our emotions and sensations, and at the same time thinking will have an impact on what we feel, our emotions and physical sensations.

Thinking is informed by feelings, and we then feel about what we think. It's not an 'either/or' situation; we do not think or feel. The healthy 'I' is holistically functioning with both. They feed each other and gain from each other.

'Intellectualising is making whatever is going on into an intellectual exercise, and as such is more often than not a form of trauma survival.

Acceptance

No one can hurt you if you see the impossibility of a situation and accept it. You cannot lose if you truly accept reality as it is.

Real acceptance cannot be faked, and can only come from the healthy 'I', and in turn it sustains and strengthens the healthy 'I'.

Real acceptance can only come when we have fully engaged with the issue, and have seen realistically and truthfully the situation as it is, and realised the impossibility of changing it. Then you are free.

The great thing about honest acceptance is that no one can hurt you. You have moved beyond being hurt.

———————∞———————

Adoption

Intention: "I want to be set free"

Adoption is, of course, an undeniable rejection by the mother and father. However, contrary to the rejection of a successful abortion, the unwanted child is permitted to live.

The child is allowed to live, but of course there are profound consequences. Below I will share what I have learned about working with different forms of adoption experience for the child.

1. Adoption immediately after birth:

If no one tells the child, as she grows up, that she was adopted, there is a deception enacted on the child. The adoptive parents know the child is adopted, and regardless of their reasons for adopting, they deceive the child every day if they do not honour the truth by telling the child at some point. Dishonesty reigns here, and the likelihood is that somewhere within the child there is an awareness of something that is not, and cannot be mentioned.

Such is the case when, during an IoPT exploratory process, the topic of the person perhaps having been adopted comes up from one of the representations, and the person says that somewhere within them they have often thought that they might have been adopted. Such a truth cannot in the end be suppressed.

The issue of whether a child is created from the sperm and egg of the parents with whom they live, or not, is a deep question in the psyche of the adopting parents. What or who do they see when they look at the child, and know, each time they see the child that she or he is not their child? In my view it is not possible for the child to live in such an environment without, probably more unconsciously than consciously, picking up some sense of something not being quite right.

If the adoptive parents decide to tell the child that she was adopted, over the time that this information sinks into the awareness of the child there are likely to come many questions and thoughts and fantasies. Questions such as "Who were my parents? Why did they have me adopted? Where are they now?" And perhaps later on the question comes as to whether it is a good idea to try and find the biological parents. Perhaps the child exists within an adoptive family where such questions can be asked, and answered honestly, and perhaps not.

From the IoPT perspective, for the child to live for nine months within the flesh of his or her mother, to have established a relationship with her (which itself must already have been traumatic), and then go through the incredibly intimate collaborative process of a vaginal birth, or, perhaps the more traumatic and choiceless (for the child) exit by Caesarean section, means that, whatever the nature of it, there is already a close relationship between the two, the mother and child. Already the child will have suffered a Trauma of Identity and a lack of a free flow of love between mother and child because the mother is intent on adoption. The child will have already established the necessary survival strategies to manage some connection with the biological mother. The primitive and vital need of the child is connection, in the form of an exchange of love, with the mother. Even after the trauma has occurred, that need is still compelling for the child, and functions throughout the pregnancy. His survival depends on it. To then be taken from her and handed to adoptive parents, no matter how loving and welcoming they are, will itself be traumatic. There is already a relationship that is now withdrawn and broken, and a new one has to be made.

During the nine-month period within the body of the mother, the state of the mother's psyche has its own impact on the child. How does a mother go through nine months of pregnancy with the constant topic of potential adoption? Is she being forced into adoption by others, her parents, or is adoption the mother's own choice? Is the pregnancy an accident, and inconvenient at the mother's time of life? Where is the father, and what is his attitude? The decision to adopt may have had to be taken over time, with much uncertainty and agony over the decision. Or it may have been made simply and irrevocably. Whatever the reasons for the mother to decide to have the child adopted, she lives through the long period of pregnancy with a living being growing inside her, drawing on her resources and emotions, living off her very flesh, blood and hormonal secretions, utterly dependent on her. Nine months is a long time to carry a child that ultimately you have decided to give away. The only possible way to do this is for the mother to make her body and her child into an object. She has to objectify the baby, and probably that part of her body that holds the baby. She has to deprive the child of his or her subjectivity, and to withdraw her own subjectivity from the child, and to an extent from herself.

The emotions of the mother during this long time feed their own hormonal effects into the child. It is all there and the child cannot avoid any of it. The mother's fear, anxiety, indecision, emotional reactions, perhaps conflictual feelings and experiences if others are involved in the decision. What of the father? What of the mother's relationship with the father? Does he agree to the adoption, or does he in fact force the issue on the mother? Or is he never consulted and never told? Are the mother's parents involved in the decision? Do others put pressure on the mother? And so on. All of this is already part of the child's existence.

The most positive thing one can say about adoption from the child's perspective really is that the child is permitted to live.

In addition, the general perception of this process is one that focuses on the mother's emotional issues, perhaps her trauma of having to give up her child. So long as the child lives and has a home to go to, little thought is given to the emotional life of the child in that moment. More often than not bonding is assumed to be a simple issue, and even seen as only relevant once the child has exited the mother's body. For the child to then bond with new parents is generally regarded as quite possible and assured.

I was invited once to give an IoPT presentation on trauma to quite a large group of gynaecologists, obstetricians, midwives and doulas, mostly women. They expressed an interest in the topic of trauma and I was excited to introduce them to basic IoPT theory.

However, I realised from the presentations that were given before mine, that the current focus of these people was the issue of trauma as it pertained to the mother during her pregnancy and birthing of her child. They were busy with thinking about how to ensure that the mother did not suffer a trauma. That was as far as their trauma awareness had got.

My presentation, of course, made the focus much more on the potential trauma of the in-utero child.

This was quite shocking for them, as they shared the common perception that the child's life in the womb is safe and untroubled by emotions and trauma. The idea that a child could suffer trauma while still within the supposed safety of the mother was completely new to them, and rather bewildering and shocking.

2. Why do mothers (and fathers) decide to give up their child?

These reasons are often complex and always highly emotional and conflictual, and also confused with the trauma survival strategies of the mother, and perhaps the father. Sometimes it is the situation that the father is not even told of the pregnancy.

Why does a mother choose adoption over abortion for example? Perhaps religious or ethical reasons, or perhaps the basic issue of the absence of safe and reliable abortion facilities, particularly if abortion is illegal in the mother's country. Or perhaps simply the unbearable notion of being responsible for killing another human being, a child. What are the conscious and unconscious hopes and fears of the mother who contemplates giving her child away? How does she organise herself to live with the issue of having given her child away?

I know of a couple who, because they were very young, and at the time unmarried, decided to have their first child adopted. I know one of them now, many, many years later, and I know that this given away child dominated their relationship, which eventually, despite their marriage and two further children that they happily kept, disintegrated into divorce. The issue of the adopted child still causes distress and sadness in the parent I know, now some 50 years on from the original adoption.

3. Why do people adopt?

There is a variety of reasons that people decide to adopt a child, and every single one of them has an impact on the child. The child is permitted to live, but is forced to live in whatever the emotional and psychological environment of the adoptive parents is, including their trauma and their own individual array of trauma survival strategies.

The most positive situation would be where the adoptive parents long for a child and are unable to conceive on their own. There is a chance in such a situation that there is love available for the child, but even so it isn't the biological mother's love; it is a substitute love.

And at the same time, the adoptive mother's loving ability will, to an extent, always be tinged with her own sorrow that the child is not hers. In effect, the presence of the adopted child is a constant, perhaps heart-breaking, reminder of the adopting mother's inability to conceive her own child. The child is a substitute child, not hers, not her flesh and blood, and she did not carry this child in her own body for the crucial nine months of potential loving and bonding. The bonding is a secondary one for child and the adoptive mother; both are suffering a substitute to what they really want. This can never be resolved. This is the price the child and adoptive mother must make for life. That is the best possible adoption solution.

From there we have to see that the survival strategies of these 'new' parents necessarily force the child into a further compromise and adaptation to a new situation. As in any other normal parental situation, the degree of healthy ability versus trauma-survival ability in these new parents has a profound influence on the child, in addition to what he or she has already had to deal with in being taken from his real mother.

A worse situation is one where the new parents are severe perpetrators, who choose to adopt from their own perpetrator instincts, and for their own survival use and exploitation. In such situations the level of perpetration towards the child can so easily escalate ... after all the child is not theirs, and therefore can be seen as available for the new parents' exploitative purposes.

Perhaps even worse is a situation where the child goes through the fostering process before finally being adopted when older, or not. Some children are forced to remain almost permanently until adulthood within a 'temporary' fostering system, never to be formally adopted. The child's survival of these terrible circumstances must involve trauma after trauma, a growing mountain of neglect and absence of any kind of real loving connection. The survival strategies for the child are so likely to slide into addictions, serious physical self-perpetration and harming, as the natural will to live and flourish is diminished by each trauma.

3. The Child's Survival Process

Knowing that he or she is adopted has a great impact on the child. What kind of relationship can develop on these terms, and what does the child do with the information that there is another mother and father whom she does not know or have contact with? There are various basic forms of this issue if the child knows he is adopted:

- Perhaps the child is the result of an unwanted pregnancy of a young girl, and the girl's family decide to adopt the child, and the actual mother becomes a 'sister' to the child and the child's grandmother is known as the mother. The adopted child is absorbed into the mother's biological family, but is confused as to who is who because no one talks about it. Such a confusing situation. There may well be benefits in the fact that at least the child is held within his biological family, but the confusion as to who is who and what the truth is will cause never-ending uncertainty in the child. Another issue is if the child, not having been born within a 'legitimate' marital relationship, is a stigma of shame for the family.
- The adopted child in a new family is told that she is adopted. This raises many questions in the child ... Why? How? Who? If the child is allowed to know her biological mother, and perhaps father, this at least provides some answers, as difficult and challenging as it may be for all concerned ... child, biological parents and adoptive parents.
- The adopted child is told by her adoptive parents that she is adopted, but the adoption was done through a system where the biological parents are to remain unknown. Even the adoptive parents do not know who the biological parents are. Some of these systems do allow for the child, upon reaching adulthood, to petition to find their biological mother, but only if the biological mother is willing. These are tricky issues, and extremely challenging for the child ... and for the adoptive parents.

Intention: "I want to be set free"

In the enquiry process with the intention above, the first thing to notice is the passive form of the intention. "to be set free" implies that someone else holds this power and authority, not the person herself. Someone else is required to set the person free. In IoPT thinking we regard this as not possible, that in order to heal our trauma we have to take responsibility for ourselves and take our trauma seriously. The notion that someone else has to do something results in a passive, inauthentic helplessness ... a victim mode of trauma survival.

As this particular process progressed the information emerged that the enquirer fell into the last category noted above: she knew she was adopted but had no idea who her biological parents were. This enquirer was new to IoPT thinking, and this process was her first attempt at setting an intention. So, as the process continued, eventually I suggested bringing in representatives for these unknown biological parents. I had not done this before, and was curious to see what would happen.

The representative for the 'biological mother' immediately started to cry and collapse. "I am so, so sad and heartbroken", and she continued to sob. Meanwhile the representative for the 'biological father' also began to cry and speak of his regret at the situation. However, one very interesting thing in the process was that these 'parents' did not seem to have any relationship with each other, they both just kept sobbing and saying how sorry and sad they were.

After watching this for a few minutes I understood the situation. These parents were a myth. They were the enquirer's creation, the parents she wished for, and yet had never known.

If we, as practitioners, understand that we are always working with representations within the psyche of the enquiring person, we can then understand that, as part of her survival construction, this woman had from very young proposed her parents to be these loving and sad parents. She had created a Reality Level 3[2] fantasy story that helped her to deal with the dilemma of her parents having given her away.

There will of course be the underlying traumas of identity and love, but at this stage of her work, this was the important point. This fact was borne out by the change in her (and her original representatives) as she understood the information. Suddenly she felt free. She had freed herself from this illusionary survival strategy. From there she is free to set further intentions to connect with the residue within her of what actually happened. A good outcome.

---

[2] Reality Level 1 is the objective world around us as it is, and our relationship to it.
Reality Level 2 is our own inner perception of Reality Level 1, which is profoundly influenced by our trauma and our survival strategies, and so, often is not commensurate with Reality Level 1.
Reality Level 3 is the delusional and illusionary constructions of our survival strategies that have no or very little relationship to Reality Level 1.

Affirmations force a fight

Intention: "I fearlessly breathe and express myself"

This intention is in the form of an affirmation.

In the world of affirmation thinking and 'therapy', an affirmation is a statement that you repeat to yourself with the idea that by doing this persistently you can make it a reality in your life. So, in the beginning an affirmation is something you tell yourself that, at that time, is not true. Whether it becomes a reality in your life, as is claimed by such therapies, or not, is up for debate, however, in IoPT thinking, affirmations become more survival strategies that distract away from dealing with the real issue, the underlying traumas.

Setting an intention in the form of an affirmation, then, is an attempt to override reality. It is a statement of defiance, to survive the helplessness of childhood, but if continued it just remains a fight against that in the person that longs for real health.

In the above intention, for example, the underlying reality is that the person cannot breathe in this way. If this were not the case there would be no point in setting the intention, because there would be no problem in the first place. So, the first thing we can know about such an intention is that, as a statement, this claim is not true. The affirmation is a false idea, a lie that one tells oneself, and then has to live up to. In this way one sets up a conflict within oneself, a split between the part that makes the claim and the part that has to be convinced. There is no good future in such a strategy.

Any statement, or intention, that falls into this category of an affirmation attempts to ignore the truth and reality, and immediately puts one in conflict with oneself. To tell myself every morning that 'I love myself', means that I try to ignore the reality of self-hatred and self-perpetration, and the underlying trauma of being the child of a hating and dismissive mother. Affirmations attempt to overlook the trauma, and as such encourage more survival strategies.

Affirmations also avoid the challenge of wanting. To really want something for oneself makes one vulnerable ... to not getting it, to being answered with a 'no', to failing. For many people, to say that they want something is, itself, a tremendous challenge. The Trauma of Identity, of not being wanted for myself, for who I actually am, requires the child to give up his wanting ability and comply with the wants of the mother, and later the father. I remember very well my mother saying to me as a child "'I want' doesn't get". For some people the ability to want something is severely prohibited, to the point where they do not allow themselves even to know *that* they want, or *what* they want. The affirmation helps to avoid the challenge of deciding for myself what I actually want, and it protects me from making myself vulnerable to not achieving my want, and perhaps even to the shame of not being able to achieve what I want. It is a statement that is not true, and the IoPT facilitator needs to be able to recognise this kind of intention.

That is not to say that it is not a valid intention. Of course, all intentions are fine, but they do show certain information by how they are formed and stated. This intention, through the representations, showed the constant fight at the beginning of life to stay alive, and, when the representative for 'breathe' said of the mother "I have to breathe her [the mother's] breath", the underlying usurping of the child's life by the mother was clear.

--------- ⌒⌒ ---------

All mothers are perpetrators

Because all mothers are traumatised ... and because all mothers' mothers are traumatised.

That seems such an outrageous and extreme thing to say. How could it possibly be true?

I'm 75 years old ... I've lived a long-ish time, and if I think back over the whole of my life, and the many, many people that I have met, known, loved and sometimes hated, I cannot think of one that I could now, with my IoPT perspective, say was not traumatised. I can see the symptoms of trauma ... I can remember the behaviours that I now recognise as the survival strategies of trauma, in all of them.

I'm not counting all the many, many psychotherapy clients I have seen over the past 30-odd years, because, after all, they are coming for help. That, in itself, means that they do not have a sufficiently healthy functioning 'I' to solve the problems of their life, and that is because of trauma, and where trauma is, there is a perpetrator mother. So, I leave out all of those who have sought me out for therapy, since it is obvious they are traumatised.

My psychotherapy trainers? Hmm. I'm not going to say anything about them, except that I am not going to count them either. They, too, showed their trauma by their choice of profession and how they lived their lives.

No, I'm thinking of all the other people I have met, friends, parents' friends, friends' parents, larger family members, teachers, fellow students, employers and employees, fellow workers, chance meetings along the way, lovers, and more lovers ... that's everybody ... not one single person could I say I didn't think was traumatised.

So, at that point I feel justified to say that all mothers are perpetrators. Certainly, I would have to say all of those people's mothers that they were all perpetrators to their children. They were traumatised themselves, of course, but for reality and truth's sake, they were all perpetrators.

We must bear the truth, because only the truth can set us free and help us live a sane life.

--------- ✿ ---------

Am I trustworthy?

The IoPT Practitioner needs to be worthy of their client's trust. There is no reason that the enquiring person should trust the practitioner, particularly if they are new to the work. The practitioner has to earn that trust.

People who come to work with us bring all their trust issues with them. Perhaps they trust too willingly, or perhaps their childhood experiences have caused them to trust no one. The IoPT practitioner can do nothing about either of these situations. The only thing the IoPT practitioner can do is ensure that they are worthy of their clients' trust, and the best way that they can do this is to be honest, and trust what is healthy in their client, *and* to trust their client's survival strategies when they come up. They come up for a reason.

Sometimes I start an exploration process session by saying quietly to myself "I trust this person knows what she is doing". That helps me to remember that somewhere in this person they do actually know what they are doing, and they also know, probably more unconsciously than consciously, how far they can go at this moment in their lives. The tension between the healthy impulse to heal oneself and the survival impulse to keep safe is always there.

People's survival strategies are their defences against what they propose to do ... to come into contact with their trauma. But ... as the person is at this moment, they are in fact doing their best under the circumstances, survival strategies and all.

To put it simply: if the person's survival strategies come up, their trust in you and the process has gone down. The more survival strategies, the less trust in the practitioner and the process, and with less trust the more the fear of going further. For the practitioner to push too much against this survival impulse puts them in danger of being the cause of an unhelpful re-traumatisation[3], and then trust is lost completely; the practitioner is the perpetrator.

In my view it is not the practitioner's job to try to eliminate or avoid or undermine or push against the person's survival strategies when they come up. They are messages from the less conscious part of the client. Perhaps the best kind of intervention here is to observe to the person the presence of their survival impulses, along with the understanding that they have come up for a reason ... and see what happens next.

---

[3] In the process of healing our trauma we do have to come into contact with our trauma, the experiences and feelings that have been split off and kept out of our daily consciousness, and we could call this a re-visiting of our trauma. For this to be useful and not unhelpful, we need to be in a good and safe environment and remain constantly aware of the strengths and resources we have, our healthy 'I', and those resources around us that we can draw on, for example in the IoPT process our representatives, the facilitator and others in the group with whom we feel safe enough. A re-traumatisation that transports us back to the original trauma moment, with a loss of connection with the here-and-now reality and the actual resources and supports that are really there now, with no good, transformative outcome is not helpful.
You might want to read my blog piece on my website: https://www.vivianbroughton.com/2017/04/24/steps-to-understanding-re-traumatisation/

A necessary digression

In nature, in mammals for instance, there is, as far as we can perceive, no 'wanting' or 'not wanting' of their offspring. Sex is an impulse of hormonal release, and mammals respond to the hormones and chemicals that arise in them, mate and produce offspring. There is no considered connection between mating and the later giving of birth and impulse to care for the young. During this process the hormones that are released prompt mother and offspring to bond, and the mother to care for the offspring, and the cubs or lambs to turn to the mother for safety and connection.

In the case of humans, with our developed psyche and consciousness, there is a 'wanting' and a 'not wanting' of the offspring. And there is the underlying issue of trauma, the traumabiography. No other species suffers trauma as we do. A primary reason for this is that the development of our intellect caused our brain to grow, which caused our skull to grow, which meant that in order to be birthed we had to be born earlier and earlier, leaving us acutely vulnerable and dependent for a considerable period of time. Our highly developed and creative intellect had a price, and that price was our vulnerability to traumatisation.

Some facts:

- 2.5 million years ago the human brain weighed 400-450 grams. Now the human brain weighs approximately 1350 to 1450 grams. The human skull has had to grow to house this enormous, and still growing, brain.
- The human head is much bigger in relation to the body than in any other species. Think of the cheetah, whose head is tiny by comparison to her body, because her body is the means of her natural survival.
- An additional stress for humans came when we began to stand upright. It helped us to develop further by leaving our hands free to manipulate our environment, but it also closed down, to an extent, the birth canal and the ability of the skeleton to expand to keep up with the growing skull of the baby.
- The evolutionary solution to this dilemma of how to birth a child whose head continues to grow and has to get through the mother's bony birth canal was to birth the offspring earlier and earlier.

- Human babies are in fact born twelve months prematurely. "Gestation should be 21 months."[4]
- Therefore, the human baby is intensely vulnerable for much longer than any other species, and so, is acutely liable to traumatisation in a way that other species generally are not.[5]
- Therefore, the mother as an adult is likely to be traumatised herself from her beginnings, and therein lies the problem: traumatised mothers traumatise their children.

I call this the 'obstetrical dilemma', the two opposing evolutionary pressures in human development resulting in the biological trade-off between the human move to stand upright, thereby constricting the further development of the pelvic structure in the female, and the continuing development of the human brain and skull. The only solution was for the baby to birth 12 months before its full time.

This leaves the human infant vulnerable in a way that no other species is. And this is why human beings are so prolifically and commonly traumatised that we have not even realised it. We regard how we are as normal, and develop philosophies and psychological ideas attempting to explain why we are the way we are, and always, until now, the topic of trauma has been in the background, regarded as unusual rather than actually as common as it is.

---

[4] Charles D. Bluestone: Humans are born too soon: impact on pediatric otolaryngology
https://pubmed.ncbi.nlm.nih.gov/15627440/ :~:text=Humans%20are%20born%2012%20months,with%20all%20of%20its%20disadvantages.

[5] I say 'generally' here because there are instances where we can see that an animal is traumatised in a similar way to our human traumatisation. But these are always circumstances that are unusual in nature and most commonly due to human intervention. An example would be the baby elephants in the elephant orphanage in Kenya, whose mothers were killed by humans for the ivory of their tusks.

Anonymity and fame

Anonymity is much more precious than fame.

That was a thought I had the other day, and it is because fame attracts perpetrators. As soon as you are famous people will envy you and try to bring you down, or they will exalt you and not see you for who you really are. It is easy to get caught in the exaltation and believe that you are greater than you are.

Anonymity is safe, simple and easy. Anonymity does not mean that your life is worthless; excellence in what you do does not necessarily bring you fame, nor does it require fame. After all, fame is all about identification. If you hanker after fame, are you not really looking for the love that you did not get from your mother?

A statement of truth

Intention: "What is that part in me that hates?"

Said in the process by the representative for the '?':

"I would rather lie down in my grave than accuse my mother, so instead I will hate myself."

A tale of two mothers ...

This is a tale of two mothers: one who exists and is traumatised, and one who never existed at all.

A message to a past lover:

"I am not your hating mother!

"Your self-hatred reflects your mother's hatred for you. She did not want you and did not love you and this is your trauma. Instead, perhaps, she hated you, but in order to survive, you, even as a baby, had to, and wanted to and needed to, have connection with her. You wanted her love, and to give her the only thing you had to give, your beautiful innocent child-love for her.

"She feared you, and her resulting hatred of you comes from her own trauma, and for you this meant that in order to have your needed contact with her as an infant, you had to align yourself with her hatred of you. So out of unconscious loyalty to your mother, who should have wanted and loved you, you had to abide by her rules, her perspective, her psychological state, and hate yourself.

"But do not include me in your psyche as also a person who hates you. I am not that mother. If I take my trauma seriously and manage to function from my healthy 'I', then I cannot be this hating mother for you. I am not her.

"On the other hand, if I do not take my own trauma seriously, and do not take steps to heal myself from my own trauma, my own disaster as a baby and child, then I, in my trauma survival capacity, can so easily become that mother for you, and hate you, and be the focus of your hatred. Together we can re-create this terrible disaster every day if we do not take ourselves and our trauma seriously."

*

"But nor am I the mother you yearn for, the mother whose love you continually long for. I cannot take that role either, because I am not her, and this mother you fantasise about did not exist. She was and is impossible. She is an illusion in the recesses of your psyche. Your mother was traumatised and used you for her own survival means, and she never was that longed-for mother. And so, I cannot be this either, this fantasised perfect, ever-loving iconic mother. If I try to fulfil this role for you I will, of course, fail, because that is not me, and you will end up hating me for failing, and I will end up hating myself for failing you."

*

"I cannot heal your trauma for you, and I cannot fulfil your fantasies. I do not want to fall into the hating mother, and I cannot be your illusionary loving mother. If I attempt to do this I will fail, and it will destroy us.

"In my healthy 'I', I love you as my lover, my partner with whom I want to share my life ... if I can stay in my healthy 'I' ... Because I, too, am traumatised, and I, too, have a real mother who did not love me and did not want me, and deep within me I also have a longed-for non-existent mother.

"We can only have a healthy relationship if we can see each other from our healthy 'I', and recognise when we lose that and collapse into our trauma survival ways. Is this in itself not enough of a reason to take our trauma seriously? I want to love you, and not miss you as you, not replace you with my traumatised fantasies and illusions, and I want the same of you. And perhaps it is in the turmoil of our relationship that we could actually find each other ... and together heal ourselves. Or perhaps it is too much for us and we have then to go our separate ways so that we do not kill each other with our self-hatred and illusionary hopes."

*

It is many years now since the relationship that triggered these thoughts. I have a wish that I had known then what I know now, and had been able to say these things. In reality it did destroy our relationship.

This is a tale of two mothers: one who exists and is traumatised, and one who never existed at all.

A university degree

When I think about 'retiring' (whatever that means!), or working less, I muse about doing a degree.

I did badly at school as a child, mostly I think out of rebellion against my father, for whom good grades and exam results and university degrees were the most important thing, and I was such a resounding disappointment to him for not being a boy, the only thing I could really do was fail in other ways, particularly academically.

Sometimes I have thought about doing a degree in psychology ...

A degree in psychology?! No ... I do not need it now I have IoPT.

Back in the '60s ...

All the protests and demonstrations, Dylan's songs about humanity, love, war and living in the world. We thought they would make a difference. We thought *we* would make a difference ... a real difference.

Perhaps we did, but it sure doesn't look like it now. The beautiful songs that Dylan wrote pleading for change ... "Come in,' she said. "I'll give ya shelter from the storm"

"How many years can some people exist, before they're allowed to be free?

Yes, and how many times can a man turn his head and pretend that he just doesn't see?

The answer, my friend, is blowin' in the wind, yes the answer is blowin' in the wind."

This cry cannot be understood, or answered, without understanding trauma.

Behind all sexual trauma is a lack of love

Intention: "I want to heal my sexual trauma"

Sexuality is about being alive, it is an expression of our life force. All species, in different ways, are entirely engaged in sex ... that is life's persistent impulse to replicate and continue itself in all its millions of different forms. All other basic needs of all species are aligned towards this furtherance of life.

If sexuality is about being alive, a primary force of existence, then we have to separate healthy sexuality from sexual traumatisation. Sexual trauma is a form of traumatisation that came through a sexual experience; but to then attempt to banish sexuality is an attempt to banish your lifeforce. Sexual trauma is a threat to life.

Behind sexual trauma is, of course, a lack of love, the Trauma of Love. The child then mistakes the sexualised attention for love.

And behind the trauma of love is the issue of not being wanted. The child can do nothing about not being wanted, but sees the issue of gaining love in the form of attention as possible if he just does whatever seems to please either of his parents. This makes him excruciatingly vulnerable to sexual exploitation by sexually traumatised perpetrator parents.

———————⟡———————

Blood pressure

It's not the high blood pressure that is the problem ...

It's the broken heart from the Trauma of Love.

Perhaps high blood pressure is a symptom of our broken heart. Set an intention to find out.

———————⟡———————

Breathing ...

... is the essence of being alive. Most of us do not breathe properly.

If we breathed properly, we would breathe right down into our diaphragm, which expands down into our lower abdomen, and we would feel it throughout our body. But to breathe properly, then, opens up our body to feeling, and that must include the split off and suppressed trauma feelings. This is why we do not breathe properly; it is the shut-down of our body in order not to feel the split off trauma feelings, the emotional pain of our trauma. Most of us breathe only into the upper part of our lungs, some almost do not breathe into the lungs at all.

We need oxygen to oxygenate the blood, and to be alive.

Watch your clients' breathing. Watch your own breathing.

Burnout ...

Trying to do the impossible ...

... in the face of constant re-triggered trauma.

Actually, burnout is a constant re-traumatisation.

Calling the mother by her name

The mother who insists that her child calls her by her first name does not want to be a mother ... she, then, obviously does not want the child.

The child wants a Mama, a Mummy, a Maman, a Mutti or whatever language fits... he does not want an Erica, or a Susan, or an Elizabeth. He wants a mother, not someone who wants to relate to him as an adult when he is so very young.

<hr />

Concepts and constructions

When we are in contact with ourselves, we don't need concepts and constructions in order to say who we are. Watch how you may wrap yourself up in ideas and constructed personas ... that is not who you are.

"I am an IoPT facilitator". Is that who I am?

<hr />

Confusion to clarity

Setting an intention is an indication of confusion, and we set intentions *because* we are confused. Confusion is the domain of the split psyche, the domain of a dominant survival mode of being. The purpose of the IoPT process is to go from confusion to clarity.

Clarity is the domain of the healthy 'I'. So, if you feel confused about anything you can know that you are in that moment functioning more from your trauma survival instincts, and the best solution then is to set an intention to resolve your confusion and gain clarity.

Confusion comes before clarity, and in a useful IoPT exploration process there should be clarity by the end. Sometimes the confusion gets worse as we go into the exploration process, but at some point, comes the clear light of clarity.

Creativity

Intention: "I want my creativity"

To be oneself and resolve one's own trauma is the most creative thing we can do.

But our creative impulse is so often put into constructing more inventive and magical survival strategies rather than resolving our trauma.

Focus your creative impulse on yourself, your real self. Who are you?

Discussion and argument ...

What is the difference?

Discussion takes place between people interested in sharing ideas in order to explore and understand something together, and perhaps find something new. It is an exchange of thoughts without the need to win. This impulse to understand together creates a win-win situation. No one is out for supremacy over the other, and so everyone wins. The interaction is a healthy 'I' to healthy 'I' meeting.

Argument is what happens between two people who are not interested in finding something new, but within themselves feel attacked and so, need to defend themselves. Argument is a survival 'I' to survival 'I' interaction, and is fuelled by the need to win ... and someone then must lose. This is the basis of perpetrator-victim dynamics.

Debate seems to me, more often than not, to be argument dressed up as discussion. Debate seems civilised, but it is about winning, and someone loses.

———————————— ᦞ ————————————

Dissociation

Intention: I want to stay associated with myself

There has been a long history of attempts to understand and define what exactly dissociation is. There is a complex article by Onno van der Hart and Rutger Horst entitled The Dissociation Theory of Pierre Janet (1989).

Pierre Janet (1859-1947) is generally acknowledged to be the originator of the 'theory of dissociation', although historically he is not the first to use the term, or to discuss what it is.

We know that dissociation is the defining symptom of traumatic experiences, but defining what exactly it is and how it works has been the subject of many definitions and much debate.

Here is my definition:

Dissociation is a separation from reality. It is the primary response to a situation that has become traumatic. If reality is too distressing, or too triggering of our unresolved trauma, then dissociation kicks in and we shut down our normal relationship with reality. It is a kind of mini psychosis that renders reality less real, and therefore less threatening.

The word 'association', in the above intention sentence "I want to stay associated with myself" then means that the person wants to stay connected with herself in whatever the current reality is; not to separate herself from herself in her experience of fear, for example.

It was from this process that I learned this definition of what dissociation is: the withdrawal from reality in the moment.

———————————— ᦞ ————————————

Disentangling myself

Intention: "Who am I?"

There are likely to be many answers to this question, so it is quite possible to set this (or any) intention several times. The primary issue we are dealing with in IoPT is the loss of self, the loss of a clear and dominant healthy 'I', and that is due to trauma, the Trauma of Identity. This then means that we do not know who we are; we have had to split and live by other's wishes and wants.

Often, particularly in the beginning of our journey to heal our trauma, the process shows, instead, "who I am *not*" This addresses the entanglements in our psyche with others, primarily our mother, but also possibly our father, and even one or other of our grandparents, and our entanglement with *their* history, *their* trauma, *their* pain. As if in some unconscious, or even conscious, part of themselves they ask us, their child, their baby, their grandchild, their responsibility, to relieve them of *their* pain, to join them in *their* pain, to save them from *their* pain, to heal them from *their* trauma.

The essence of the Trauma of Identity is that we cannot hold onto our separateness. Surviving requires us to adapt and compromise, to give up on ourselves as a separate and autonomous being, and instead our survival requires us to merge, identify, adopt the ways and wants of the perpetrator. The infant cannot resist or fight the perpetrator; his vulnerability does not offer the necessary resources to hold onto himself and his own 'I'. He has no intellect to even understand the problem ... he is an organism without sufficient means to make sense of what is happening ... all he knows is he has to do whatever it takes to survive. Life's primary impulse is to stay alive if possible.

So, these entanglements are deeply unconscious, having been established long before we have the intellect to understand what is happening, and in the intention process there is the possibility of a freedom just to see these entanglements and to realise at the first level, "I am not these people".

"I am not my mother; I am not my father; and I am not my grandmother". This strengthens and clarifies, then, who I actually am.

As we continue our work, the depth of the entanglement, particularly with our mother, becomes increasingly obvious. Then it is not enough to say "I am not my mother". Instead, I begin to see how much the entanglement with her means to me, how much I hold onto her, even as an adult, even as an avid student of IoPT theory ... I still hold onto the threads of connection, no matter how much this harmed me and continues to harm me. The longing for her endures, and I then remain entangled.

The original entanglement was forced on us. The here-and-now entanglement is not. In the beginning we could do nothing; we had no resources, no defence against this take-over, this invasion of our psyche by the person who is most important in our world. But now, as adults, no one forces this on us; we do it to ourselves. We keep our perpetrator and invading mother in our psyche ... no one else does this to us anymore.

Here are two questions:

> *How* do I keep my mother in my psyche?
> *Why* do I keep my mother in my psyche?

Becoming increasingly conscious of how I hold onto this entanglement as an adult is hard, and painful, because it is only when I really see and feel the underlying pain of not being loved, of not being able to hold onto myself and my wants, of in effect being robbed of myself and my wants, that I can then begin to disentangle myself. The longing for our mother's love transcends many of our healing attempts. It is not easy to relinquish this child longing within us.

———————— ⌁ ————————

"Don't feed me to your mother!"

Intention: "I want to stop obeying mama"

The 'I' representative to the enquiring person: "I will belong to you so long as you don't keep feeding me to your mother."

———————— ⌁ ————————

Enter the perpetrator ...

Where there is a problem in our life that we cannot solve by ourselves, there is trauma. Problems can be solved when we are in our healthy 'I' state, and if there is no feasible solution, we can see this too from our healthy 'I' perspective. But if we stay with a problem and cannot resolve it, that is because it puts us in touch with our trauma, sending us into our splits and our survival 'I'. Then we can understand that whatever the 'problem' is, the fact that we cannot resolve it is due to trauma.

And where there is trauma, there is a perpetrator.

A primary question for the IoPT facilitator, from the moment the process starts, can be: where do I see the perpetrator?

The primary trauma that underlies all other traumas is what we in IoPT have called the Trauma of Identity, and this is the traumatisation of the child by the mother, by her not wanting her child. In the actual process, of course, depending on what topic the person wants to address, may show another perpetrator, the father for instance, or another perpetrator from later in life ... but underlying all later traumas is this Trauma of Identity, and that trauma is perpetrated by the mother. So, the primary perpetrator is always the mother.

The perpetrator will be there, in the enquiry process, in one of the representatives, but also, perhaps, in the enquiring person him or herself. After all, the Trauma of Identity requires the child to align herself with her mother, and her mother's wants, wishes, prejudices and behaviours. The enforced alignment then means that the child will come to behave towards herself as her mother behaves towards her. "My mother hates me; therefore, I have to hate myself." "My mother criticises me, so I criticise myself." "My mother wishes I did not exist, so I cannot exist in any meaningful way." "My mother harms and hurts me, and I, then, harm and hurt myself."

Then, comes the question: do we bring in a representative for this perpetrator who is already embedded in the process?

To bring a representative for the mother into the process is in order to gain some clarity, some distance from her; to see how the mother we keep in our psyche dominates us. The danger of bringing in a representative for the mother is that in the process she may come to dominate, and her story, her trauma takes over. This is not the point of bringing in the mother representative. Yes, perhaps some information emerges about the context in which the enquiring person arrived in the world, how the mother 'takeover' was, but this mother representative cannot be the source of healing. The impulse to talk to her, to explain ourselves to her, change her, to find the mythical loving mother, is strong in the enquiring person, and this can lead to distractions with *her* trauma and *her* story.

The mother representative is brought in to give information … hopefully useful information. She is a representative. So long as we resist owning and feel the deepest heartfelt pain that she is not, could not ever be, and will not ever be the person we long for, we keep her close, embedded in our psyche and in every moment of our life.

It makes no difference if, as an enquirer setting an intention, we tell the mother representative to go, to turn off her screen (in an online event) or get out of the role; if we continue to hold onto the underlying hope that we can get her to love us, we continue to hold her in our psyche.

Franz Ruppert suggests the solution for the person is to say to their 'I': "I long for my mother's love".

The suggested sentence is in the present tense, and is intended to deal with the present, here-and-now persistent longing, and as such, if said sincerely and with contact, will bring the person in connection with their deepest heart pain of the truth of the mother's lack of love and wanting of the child. It is only this that will allow a step towards a clearer psyche, towards a psyche no longer dominated by the mother's influence. If we go to this deep pain, we are then free to choose ourself, rather than remain split between our desire to be truly who we are and our desire for our mother's love.

I have also noticed how often this suggested sentence is taken by the person from the present form and put into the past form, as in "I *longed* for my mother's love." Put this way gives some distance from the here-and-now reality as shown in the intention process, and as such is a survival impulse. The intention process reflects the present continuing existence. To put this sentence in the past does not recognise the currency of the situation, the present here-and-now nature of the issue, and in that sense, it offers a survival distancing.

We keep our mother in our psyche. We continue to direct our love to her, and to be ruled by this mythical mother in our psyche. So long as the perpetrator takes space in our psyche, we do not truly have ourselves. The real mother is out there, living her life as best she knows how. It doesn't matter in the end who she is or who she was, nor does it matter in the end what she did or what she does, so long as we hold her there, in our psyche, the longing for her persists, and we, then, are the perpetrator to ourself.

Everyone ignores the traumatised child

That is the nature of trauma ... everyone avoids the trauma, and in the IoPT process it is easier, and safer, for the enquiring person to stay with those representatives that are showing survival strategies, and avoid the representative that is holding the trauma.

This is a parallel with what actually happened. The child is traumatised *because* he was ignored, since he was not wanted and not loved ... and he is ignored *because* he is traumatised. After all, for the perpetrator parents, the existence of a troublesome traumatised child requires some explanation, and one solution is to ignore the child. Another solution is to make the child the problem, and then of course the parents can see themselves as innocent, and as victims of this troublesome child.

The child is also ignored because it was likely to have been safer for him to be ignored. What a terrible dilemma for a child who only wants to be seen and loved, to have to find safety by making himself unseen.

The IoPT facilitator can bear this in mind and, during the IoPT process, watch for the representative that is ignored or not favoured by the enquiring person and, perhaps, the other representatives. In the physical 'in-person' process this might be the representative who hides in a corner or under a chair in a far corner of the room. In the online process it might be the one who makes themselves invisible on the screen, or even turns off their video.

The IoPT facilitator needs to try not to fall into this trap and ignore the traumatised child in their work with the enquirer's process. The ignored representative holds the solution.

Experience is about being ...

... and doing is the active expression of being.

*

Intention: "I want to experience the world as myself"

My comment on the intention:

If you are truly yourself, how can you do anything other than experience the world as yourself? You cannot experience the world as anyone else. But it is also true that in order to experience the world clearly you do need to have some sense of who you really are, to exist as yourself, not as any construction of yourself, not as your survival strategies, and definitely not as your mother's experience of herself and her life.

The intention indicates that your own experience is taken over, superseded, co-opted, consumed, stolen by the perpetrator ... your mother. Then you cannot experience the world as yourself. That is a Trauma of Identity.

First you need to come to know who you are, which means expanding and strengthening your healthy 'I', and confronting the truth of your traumatisation by your mother.

———————o√o———————

Explaining yourself

When you explain yourself to someone else, you are wanting that person to see you and validate you and your experience. That is identification, the survival strategy for the Trauma of Identity and the Trauma of Love.

Underneath your desire for the other person to hear your explanation of yourself, you are wanting your mother to see you and love you, to validate you, your experience and your existence. Everyone in your life, then, becomes your mother.

Any time you find yourself explaining yourself to anyone, think about this ... are you trying to gain your mother's love? The impulse to explain yourself may be a symptom of the Trauma of Identity and the Trauma of Love.

Facing the truth

"The truth will set you free, but first it will piss you off!"

(Gloria Steinem)

When we face the truth ...

... it strengthens us and our healthy 'I'.

But first it often brings up anger and rage against the perpetrator, and even against the 'unfairness of life', which of course is a myth. Life has no sense of justice or fairness; these are human constructs.

However, to stay with this railing against the truth is not, in the end, of any use, and does not set us free. The anger and rage may make us feel more powerful, less helpless and vulnerable, but it also is a myth, and must pass or we stay entangled and trapped, and regardless of the feeling of power that anger gives, we remain helpless.

To be angry with someone always requires something from that person ... to be heard, acknowledged, recognised, affirmed that we exist ... We remain reliant on the other, or others, to validate our existence. We demand something... perhaps acquiescence from the other, admission of guilt, of perpetration against us. Anger wants to win, and winning means someone must lose and there, already, are the dynamics of perpetration and victimisation.

Whereas anger and rage cause the body to tense up, fists to form and energy to rise, the truth relaxes the tensions in our body and strengthens our resources. Acknowledging the truth brings you back to yourself, and leaves the other to themselves.

So, you have to get past the "piss you off" phase, face the truth calmly and then you are free.

Falling into the soup

"One of our greatest freedoms is how we react to things."

(Charles Makesy, 2022)

Getting caught up in perpetrator-victim dynamics is like falling into a vast pan of blended soup. It's thick and gloopy; you can't swim and you can't get out. You can't distinguish any more what is what, carrots from cabbage ... soup is in your eyes so you cannot see, and you *are* the soup too ... so you cannot tell where you end and anyone else begins. Any attempt at differentiation ups the ante, ups the stakes.

Once caught in perpetrator-victim dynamics, our access to our healthy 'I' is seriously diminished, and we are in trauma survival; we too are perpetrator and we are victim.

Anyone who has suffered a trauma, no matter how long ago, is vulnerable to these dynamics. Whether the starting point is an altercation with a less-than-helpful storekeeper, or the invasion of one's country by another ... once the energy of the engagement is up and running all are in the soup; it is hard to stay out. It's hard to stay out because we, too, are traumatised and have within us a victim version and a perpetrator version of trauma survival strategies.

Watch your reactions to what happens in your life; notice the rise in energy, the impulse to hit back, to retort in kind, the irrepressible urge to say "Yes, but ..." and attempt to explain yourself, to uphold your rights, to demand justice. All of these are the signs that you are in danger of slipping into the soup of P-V dynamics; one more step and you are in.

Our reactions to what happens in our world tell the tale. What happens is what happens, but it is our reactions that catch us, and lure us into the soup.

All traumatised people are excruciatingly vulnerable to falling into the soup.

———— ⌀ ————

Finding the gap

"There's always a gap"

Miranda Allen, escape artist

Of course, there must be a gap for an escape artist. It isn't a magic trick. True escapology is an art; it is a skill, but it isn't magic.

I heard Miranda Allen on the radio talking about her act, and, for example, how she had trained herself to be able to hold her breath for over four minutes. Her most famous act is being chained up with heavy chains and padlocks and getting into a large wooden barrel of red wine, which is then chained up with the lid in place and a strong lock on the top. That is where she needs to be able to hold her breath, being immersed in red wine long enough to escape. You can see her perform her 'wine barrel' act on YouTube.

During the interview I had many thoughts about trauma; primarily how being drawn to being an escape artist might have parallels with the need to escape her family. Fairly obvious thoughts really.

What on earth, I thought, would make someone want to become an escape artist? Listening to her talk was very interesting, as well as her accounts of contact with members of the audience, understanding what happens to the audience, the thrill and anxiety of watching her show, what it brings up for people.

All very interesting from an IoPT perspective, but the thing that buzzed for me was when she said this thing: "There's always a gap. You just have to find the gap, and then when you find it you follow it, and the gap gets bigger."

Of course, I realised what she meant was that in all the tying up with the chains and everything else there is always a gap, a small place of looseness, some place you can use, get into, enlarge, slip along and make bigger until you can slip something through, loosen more, and eventually slip out.

Immediately it made me think of our work. Where is the gap? The gap that allows for a loosening of the tight survival construction and holding prison of the start of our life?

*

Intention: "I want to value my work well"

I was supervising a senior student facilitating a one-to-one process. The enquirer chose to resonate with the words 'I', 'work' and 'well".

Of course, as is usually the case, the process of resonance went to a young place, with the word 'work' feeling like a child being held down. As a facilitator, of course I had speculations and hypotheses as to what this might be ... but the most interesting part of the process was when the enquirer resonated with the word 'I'.

Since it was an individual session, the enquirer was doing his own resonating, and he left the word 'I' to last. To start with it was obvious that, as the 'I', he wanted not to be in contact with himself ... there seemed to be no possibility of contact between the enquirer and his 'I'. "We cannot look at each other."

And then, while still resonating with the word 'I', he came into an intriguing split: one half of him as the 'I' wanted to write, with his right hand, and wanted to write 'the truth', what he was avoiding knowing. The other half of him as the 'I', the left side, put his left hand over his eyes so he would not see what his right hand was wanting to write; this part did not want to know. The 'I' was split. There he was, resonating in his own work, and experiencing in his own body the complete impasse within him of the part of him that wants the truth to come out, and the part of him that doesn't want to know, wants to avoid and suppress the reality underlying everything.

Watching him it was easy to see the power of the energetic impasse; equal force on either side with no perceivable way out. Just like being trapped in a large barrel of red wine while wrapped in chains and heavy padlocks.

So, where was the gap? And, more than that, what then is the job of the IoPT facilitator?

There are two things here. One is an important issue about the function of the IoPT facilitator. It is tough sometimes, as a facilitator, to watch someone sit in this kind of impasse, particularly if you have a hunch as to what the underlying (and so, efficiently avoided) issue is. It is tempting to say what you think the issue is and see what happens, and many of us do so in such a situation. But is this the best thing to do?

A guiding principle throughout my psychotherapy career has been something the Gestalt therapist Fritz Perls said: "If you [the therapist] tell the person [client] something, you rob him of the opportunity to find it for himself" - or something like that. I read it years ago in one of

Perls' books, but can't find it anymore, but that was the gist of the quote. What I think about this is as follows: if there is such a strong attitude of resistance to knowing a truth in the person himself, who am I to rob him of his journey of self-discovery? Who am I to undermine his own strength of avoidance and survival? If I tell him what I think, what my hypothesis is, is that not an act of perpetration? A 'rescue' attempt? An "I know the answer" (and even an "aren't I clever?") moment?

Well, of course I have done this myself many times, but I do also, at times, feel an underlying discomfort of perhaps having crossed a boundary uninvited. As an overall principle I believe in respecting people's survival strategies; after all these strategies of avoidance were developed to protect, and who am I to decide that this act of self-protection is now out-dated and should be confronted? These are complex questions for the IoPT facilitator.

I have always seen survival strategies in the intention enquiry process as useful information as to how the person is doing, information that is best highlighted and acknowledged rather than thought of as a nuisance. We all make our own decisions as practitioners in such situations, and I, too, sometimes decide one way and sometimes the other. It is hard to watch someone else's struggle and not follow the entirely human urge to be helpful.

The second thing is: where, then, is the gap? And how to develop, loosen, extend the gap to free oneself from the barrel?

In the process I mentioned above, as the enquirer sat with this terrific dilemma, I, as the supervisor, so merely an observer, could see that in the moment the supervisee-facilitator was to some degree at a loss as to what to do next, or how to intervene or help. I could feel it myself. And, also, the entirely human instinct to want to help the student out!

And then, in a moment of complete autonomy and inspiration the enquirer spoke as himself and said: "The only thing that is important is my 'I'. Whatever I want, I need to start with my 'I'." And in that moment the tension dissolved and the client relaxed in his body and the image of the split 'I' was gone. He took the marker with his own name and the marker with the 'I' and stuck them both on himself. "I cannot do anything without my 'I'. I cannot face the truth without my 'I', without good contact with my 'I'.

He did it himself. He found his own gap and slipped into it to free himself of his conflict!

Following the narrative

Intention: "I want my memories"

One way of thinking about the IoPT exploration process as a practitioner is to follow the narrative. Often the process from the start develops as a narrative over time.

This was a process where I was supervising and supporting the IoPT practitioner who was facilitating.

The enquirer said that she had very little memory of her childhood ... she knew that there were awful things that had happened to her, but she couldn't remember them.

The first moment of such a narrative is often when one representative describes their experience as being in the womb. The representative may say that he or she feels like they are in the womb, or they may not. But the experiences expressed one could hear as 'womb-like' experiences.

In this process the 'I' started off by saying that she felt very young, in the womb. "I am swimming in water ... I am very content. I am swimming in water ... there is nothing else. I am alive and I feel good."

Immediately we can understand that this representative at this moment is before the first trauma happened. She feels good and content. She is also swimming freely in the water; in other words, the tiny infant has not yet found a place in the womb of the mother to connect and embed herself. She is free, separate, and content and happy. This newly created being is unique, independent and full of life's promise.

It may seem paradoxical when we know we are dealing with trauma to find that one of the representatives expresses their experience in this way, but there *is* a time before the trauma hits us, and this seems to me a good description of that time. We can also know by this related experience that the topic, the intention, in some way goes back to this very early stage, and it is important for the person to know that this, too, is one of her memories ... a time before the trauma. It opens up the idea that some memories are good and supportive!

The representative for 'memories' had quite a different experience: "I don't feel much ... I don't feel anything. I am in my head ... I don't understand the word 'feel'. I like your sweet face [to the enquirer] but that makes me feel a bit sad. There is a jumble in my head ... many memories, it's chaos, I feel like the top of my head is blowing off. I feel nothing from the top of my head down, and my head is in chaos ... too many things going on."

At this point the enquirer mentions something about her body, and 'memories' says "that puts me in panic ... the idea that I have a body ... I can't breathe ... my breathing might stop. Now I am semi-conscious, there's nothing ... I'm drifting."

And the 'want' said she felt separate from everyone, very small and sad.

After this the 'I' experience is quite different; she is angry, saying that "my safe space was knocked off", so in terms of the narrative we can understand that now trauma has happened ... her "safe space" has been knocked out and she is not safe anymore.

The process continued with no positive result and eventually reached a place of impasse. The 'I' was "full of anger" and 'memories' felt semi-conscious, alone, drifting (dissociated) and unable to breathe.

This is often a point where the facilitator may suggest bringing in other representatives, the mother perhaps ... a possible twin was mentioned, and, because underneath everything the issue of sexual abuse as being part of the forgotten memories was mooted, the father was also mentioned.

At this point, however, I understood three things:

1. For the enquirer to have her memories at this moment was too much. The chaos that 'memories' talked about indicated that there were many awful memories to be considered.
2. One reason that retrieving her memories was too much was because she did not have sufficient healthy 'I' strength. She did not have a connection with her 'I'. At one point the 'I' had said to the enquirer "I don't know you; I don't know who you are."
3. The original experiences related by the 'I' were, indeed, themselves memories; there is then, in her repertoire of memories, also this wonderful 'paradise' moment before the 'fall' of traumatisation.

Since at this moment the facilitator asked me in for support and suggestions, I felt free to say these three things to the facilitator, which of course the enquiring person could hear.

Immediately the enquirer turned to her 'I' who also turned towards her and there followed some moments of exquisite contact and loving feelings between them. They had come into good contact, and the session ended here.

We cannot go into the awful traumatic memories of our childhood if we do not have sufficient internal resources; our survival strategies will not allow it. We need some good contact with our 'I' as the main source of strength in order to deal with such traumas and memories, otherwise we will just overwhelm ourselves, re-traumatise ourselves, because in that moment we do not have the resources to deal with what is happening. Good contact with a healthy 'I' is a precious resource to help us on this journey.

I relate this process to you to give some idea of the sense of sequence and narrative that often happens in the process, where the 'I' started before the trauma and then was after the trauma. It also shows the logic of us: we do not remember memories if, in our current state, it would overwhelm us. Therefore, in this process two vital things happened: the feeling of a good memory and a reclaiming of connection with the 'I'. From there it becomes more possible to confront the later traumas, and eventually the earlier traumas of identity that underlie the later traumas.

We need good contact with a resourceful 'I' to confront our traumas.

Going to the movies

What makes Michael Corleone ...[6] a character that, despite his continual descent into terrible perpetration, come across as somewhat sympathetic to the audience? To take in the extraordinary massacre he organises while he himself is in church acting as godfather at the baptism of his sister's child, and then to see his supposed loving contact with his wife when his own bedroom is shot up by others, seduces us into finding him a somewhat sympathetic character.

Watching this with my IoPT thinking makes me realise this character is a fantasy. Much of what we see in our entertainment is in fact fantasy, with often only a slim relationship with reality. It is just not possible for someone who has become such a perpetrator to feel any real loving feelings towards his wife.

However, it is also true, we can see from the film, that Michael is extremely controlling of his wife and children. No real love there then. The clash of these behaviours with the attempt to show him as loving is exactly the kind of fantasy that much of our world supposes is possible, but the IoPT-informed person may recognise this fantasy for what it is.

I have watched the Godfather films many times ... they are an intriguing entertainment, at once horrifying (who can forget the horse's head in the bed sequence, and the brilliantly filmed baptism massacre?), and at the same time attempting to show a kind of humanity and attitude that draws us in.

In The Godfather II we see Robert Di Niro as the young Vito Corleone, capable of murder, and yet at the same time capable of what we would call a healthy 'I' attitude to others. When the local Italian overlord, Don Fanucci, coerces the store keeper to take on his nephew as an employee, forcing the store keeper to sack Vito, he, Vito, takes it with generous equanimity and understanding, and even refuses the store keeper's offer of a large basket of food as recompense. How do we reconcile these two seemingly unreconcilable attitudes? How do we reconcile the older (Marlon Brando) Vito Corleone happily supporting the brutal beheading of the beloved stallion of the film producer, with his tenderness towards his grandson just before his death? Is this real? Can we honestly think that real love is possible in these overwhelmingly

---

[6] From the film The Godfather I and II.

perpetrator characters? Or are we being seduced in the film into accepting the unacceptable, the murder and mayhem on all sides?

Perhaps defenders of this story would ask us to see that there is a code of humanity within the perpetration involved. "It's not personal ... it's only business" is often used in the films to justify actions, but frankly that's rubbish. It's all personal. It's just an excuse to allow for the extreme perpetrator actions. To say that it's only business when someone betrays some else, or has them murdered is completely the thinking of the perpetrator.

And the crying babies ...

Have you ever noticed how often babies in films are portrayed as crying? Here is a baby, and in order that we really know it's a baby, it must be crying ... and more than that, no one ever seems to think that the baby's crying means anything. That's just what babies do! And it is rare in films that anyone does anything about the crying baby.

The Godfather films are full of crying babies, desperately crying babies; painfully crying ... real babies. These babies are not actors acting; they are really crying. No one asked them if they were willing to be in the film, and everyone wants them to cry ... and of course they do. They have been wrested away from their mother, who is the one who decides her baby can do this acting job, perhaps for a good amount of money. No one in the films does anything for the baby; everyone seems to see this as normal, and no one ever does anything to try and understand what the crying baby is trying to communicate.

These kinds of films, the Godfather films, are indicators of where we are in our evolution as humans: blind to the reality of perpetrator-victim dynamics, and blind to the reality of trauma. If the films would make a statement about perpetrator-victim dynamics, really, without the fantasy element that a person can perform horrible acts of perpetration and still have the ability of real love and care, then we will have moved to an IoPT-informed society.

I still find the Godfather films intriguing, but increasingly hard to watch. I now have to fast-forward over the violence and the crying babies. I guess that says something about my developing healthy 'I'.

Hate and climate change

I don't think we talk about hate enough; we are too enamoured with our illusions of love. And yet the Trauma of Identity and the Trauma of Love are symptoms of hatred, sufficient to desire or wish the non-existence of the child, and then the potential hatred of the child's continued existence.

And we are currently struggling against the most calamitous symptom of our collective self-hatred and hatred of others, of trauma, the dilemma of climate change. Is not our careless exploitation of our environment the clearest symptom of trauma? Of course, all species attempt to adjust their environment to suit their needs, it's just that we have more than adjusted ... we have overtaken our environment, and subjected it to a careless and short-sighted manipulation and exploitation. We are at a crossroads: are we going to take down ourselves, our environment and all other species with us, or do we have sufficient will and clear sight to adjust ourselves?

"Inertia and optimism are powerful forces ... Nobody wants what's coming, so nobody wants to see what's coming."

(S. Marche, 2022)

The problem for us is that the issue of climate change terrifies us; it makes us feel helpless, and that re-stimulates our own trauma and, because we feel overwhelmed by our unresolved trauma feelings, we have to look away, ignore, deflect and distract. *"Nobody wants what's coming, so nobody wants to see what's coming"*. And this is what we have always done with our own private trauma, and this is what we are likely to do around this massive issue of climate change.

Think for a moment of the generations and generations of traumatised humans, making wars, persecuting others, hoarding wealth, exploiting fellow humans, enslaving our brothers and sisters, sexually traumatising children, persecuting those who do not think as we do, killing in the name of 'good', creating belief systems to justify our perpetration of others who we deem as different, inferior, alien, even evil. For over 3,000 years we have blamed women for a condition labelled hysteria (the 'wandering womb', but really a cover term for mis-understood emotionality and trauma) in order to avoid the topic of trauma, which only became a topic for study in the mid-1800s, and even today is still considered by many with suspicion, or used randomly as a word to cover any challenging situation. That diagnosis of 'hysteria' not only played into the supposed 'patriarchy' by seeing women as vulnerable and tending to irrationality, but also put on hold any consideration of the continual perpetration of trauma for many generations. That in itself is an act of hatred and indifference, subverting, as it does, the seriousness of the real issue of the traumatised mother and the resulting trauma of the unwanted and unloved child.

We have known about the issue of climate change for over a century, in fact the year of 1896 is often quoted as the time when the issue of CO_2 and potential global warming first surfaced, but the issue we are currently dealing with is our failure to do anything about it as we slide ever faster towards a drastically hotter and less viable world for us and most other species to survive within. How else can we see our continued exploitation of the resources of our world, with little thought for the resulting devastation of the environment, not just for ourselves, but for all the millions and millions of other species that our failure to act may harm and force to extinction, than at the very least as insensitive, and more accurately as the symptom of our hatred and self-hatred, as a symptom of trauma?

Our ability to kill and exploit our world without care is, in my view, a vast symptom of our ability to hate, and hatred is a symptom of trauma, and still, to an extent, we are avoiding this topic. To perform acts of destruction, or neglect the required acts of creation and preservation, is a symptom of our own attitude towards ourselves as much as towards our environment. Does not the notion of 'living a good life' include responsible caretaking of our environment? After all what does it mean to live a good life for ourselves if we destroy the environment on which we depend and in which we live that life?

As much as healing trauma means psychological and emotional healing, it also means respecting and taking care of our physical body in which we live. Care for the psyche and not the body doesn't make sense, and in the same way, care of ourselves without care for our environment also doesn't make sense. The physical symptom, whatever it is, is a symptom of something, and when we set an intention about a physical symptom, we see that it points directly to our trauma. So, in the same way I am saying that we can see our collective failure to act in terms of climate change as a symptom of trauma and as such a symptom of our collective self-hatred and self-rejection, our own personal trauma.

That does not mean that we should rush to protest, or to attempt to fix the external; we cannot properly do something about the external if we are not in good contact with our healthy 'I'; we will just get caught up in the perpetrator-victim dynamics that prevail. It has to start with the individual and a sincere commitment to oneself and to relieving oneself of one's own trauma, and developing a clear-thinking and healthy, resourceful 'I'. Maybe as a species we will fail, but we humans are also immensely creative and inventive, and a clear 'I' is the most creative possibility we have. We can only see a good way forward for ourselves from a healthy 'I' ... then we can see what is actually possible for us, and know with clarity what is not.

In my view the development of IoPT, with its understanding of the dynamics of trauma, is a major contribution to the current dilemmas we face. It offers an explanation of, and perhaps some solution to and escape route from, the chaos and dangers of our world, but it also shows us that the only solution is to look within and heal ourselves.

This leads to the next essay: Hate comes where hate is ...

———————— ⟶⟵ ————————

Hate comes where hate is ...

What is hate? Is it, for example, the opposite of love?

Where love exists, there can be no hate, and where hate exists there is no love.

The newly created child has no reason to have the experience of hate. As a newly created organism, he is only interested in the life affirming emotion and energy of love. It is the existence within him and within his mother of love that he needs in order to grow and develop into a healthy child and adult. Love is the emotion that holds him in the initial time of his existence in the womb, if it is there in his mother for him. If not, this tiny developing being is at a loss. It is the love potential that he holds within him that needs to make a loving connection with his mother, as soon as possible. Perhaps we could say that to really live one's life in a healthy way we need love, and if it does not come from our mother, we have to compromise ourselves, split off our loving ability, and bury our consistent and persistent need and yearning for love from her deep within ourselves.

This 'buried loving ability' crushes our healthy ability to love ourselves, and thence compromises our ability to love another. We end up in a sea of delusions of love that avoid the reality: where there is hatred, love is not possible.

The child only knows hate when he is hated, and once the hating door is opened, the child then knows hate, and if he received hatred from his mother he becomes well acquainted with self-hatred, and this, then, becomes the connection between them, and the state from which he lives his life.

Healing the world

This is not a truth, but it is a possibility. Theoretically it would take three generations to heal the world.

Just three generations would make the world an infinitely better place, if IoPT-informed. The topic of trauma becomes more mainstream, and each generation becomes more familiar with the impact of trauma and the individual healing impulse becomes more embedded and normal in society.

Generation 1:

This is our generation ...

- Recognises trauma, and works to heal their own trauma and clear their psyche of invasive external material, thereby ...
- Creating a clearer space for their contact with their (already traumatised) children, and ...
- Demonstrating to these already traumatised children that healing is possible, and ...
- Supporting their already adult children to heal themselves

- Accepting and acknowledging responsibility for their perpetration towards their children when appropriate, i.e., if the children ask and require it.
- Friends and colleagues notice the differences in you and the topic becomes more widely spread.

Generation 2:

- Trauma becomes a much more mainstream topic.
- This generation is already much more familiar with IoPT trauma theory, and accepts this reality
- These young adults are encouraged by their parents and other adults to take the necessary steps to heal themselves of their trauma caused by the parents
- They become IoPT-informed
- This generation then have their own children.

Generation 3:

- These children are more likely to be wanted, loved and kept safe, and ...
- Encouraged to be who they really are, and loved for that
- They are more likely to be able to grow in an environment that is based on reality, truth, honesty and trust ...
- ... where any acts of perpetration are acknowledged and amended for appropriately as soon as possible

You may say this is a fantasy, and perhaps to think that three generations is enough is a fantasy. Perhaps it will take five generations, or ten, but IoPT thinking is in the world now, and the world cannot remain the same.

———— ०‍৲০ ————

Helpful Words from 'The Godfather'

"Never hate your enemies; it affects your judgement"

Michael Corleone says this in the film Godfather III.

If you are full of hatred, you are in survival; and if you are in survival, your judgement is impaired.

You can only have good judgement when you have the clear thinking of your healthy 'I', and we do not hate from our healthy 'I'.

Surprising to find such a useful quote from such a violent and perpetrator-oriented story!

———————————— ✒ ————————————

Hope keeps us alive … and it kills us

I do not know what else to say about this … yes, hope does keep us alive as a traumatised child; the hope that perhaps one day, if I get my behaviour and existence right, my mother will see me and love me. But to keep hoping as an adult, in the face of incontrovertible evidence that the hoped-for situation is not real and will not happen, well … then it kills us.

———————————— ✒ ————————————

I abandon myself ...

... for the love of my mother

Intention: "I abandon myself"

No one naturally abandons themselves. That is against the basic impulse of nature. To abandon oneself is a split: I leave myself. Why would this be? It is not natural for any healthy being to attempt to leave itself.

So, then we have to ask the question: What does this mean for this person?

The only reason one would abandon oneself is because the mother did not want the person as a child ... therefore one has to abandon oneself ... for the love of the mother.

"I am traumatised"

This is the first statement one has to make on this journey. This is a statement of acknowledgement of a truth, and from here we can take a good step towards doing something about it.

Just to say "I am traumatised" is itself a major achievement. One may not really know what this means at the time, but the sincere acknowledgement is profound, and is the start of one's journey to health and happiness.

From this admission then arises the question: "What then should I do about it?" Well, something more is required, that is for sure.

It is a starting statement, but it is not the ending statement.

If the process gets stuck

There are occasions where the IoPT enquiry process seems to get stuck, and the representatives and the enquirer cannot find a way to come together, and the facilitator, too, cannot find a way to help them find a resolution.

In such a situation, it helps for the IoPT facilitator to remember that in *all* families there are things that it is forbidden to talk about. And, to talk about these things will bring up in the enquiring person the challenge of speaking out that which is forbidden. To speak out brings up strong feelings in the enquiring person of potentially betraying the family and the mother, with the resulting loss of any hope of gaining love from the mother. The family is a system that has strict, unspoken, rules about what can be a topic to be spoken, and what must never, ever, be touched on, what should be forgotten and never addressed.

This presents a challenge to the enquiring person, and to the facilitator.

It is often the case that the facilitator, and perhaps even one of the representatives, has a subtle sense of what it is that cannot be spoken, and both may be presented with a question as to whether to say it or not.

For myself, as a facilitator, I would always prefer that the unspoken and forbidden information comes from the process, either from a representative or from the enquiring person herself.

The question as to whether the facilitator can speak out here is complex, and needs careful consideration before doing so. After all, if we understand the function of survival strategies as the ways in which the person protects themselves, then we might think "who am I to step over that boundary?" But then, on the other hand, as the facilitator, we might see our function as to be the person who *can* say the unsayable in the absence of any of the representatives, or the enquiring person himself saying it.

Unfortunately, I cannot give you any definitive answer to the question as to what you, as a facilitator, should do in such a situation. What I am doing here is attempting to show you the issue, and what you might want to consider when you find yourself in such a situation.

A third, and perhaps preferable, option for the facilitator is to observe aloud that the stuckness that seems to exist at this moment in the process might indicate that there is something at this point that cannot be said, and see what happens.

In my view, a process that cannot continue because some vital bit of information is missing, may be eased by having this fact out in the open. Just to acknowledge that there may be something missing can either support a representative to speak out, or it may just allow for some relaxation and acknowledgement, and help to find some resolution at this time. Raising the possibility of missing information may also have an impact on the enquiring person after the process is finished.

The reality is that, in the end, the situation will not resolve until what is underneath ... pointed to in the process, but not said ... is spoken. The splits will remain.

--------⌒⌇⌒--------

"I help my clients ...

... and that makes me feel good!"

Why do we become therapists, or IoPT practitioners? If, as the quote above implies, we gain some feeling of satisfaction from helping others perhaps we need to question ourselves. Am I working as a therapist or IoPT facilitator in order to feel good about myself in the absence of such good feeling otherwise? If so, we are in danger of exploiting our clients, using them in the same way, perhaps, as our mother used us, to help us feel better about ourselves.

What is the benefit to us of working as an IoPT practitioner? If the benefit to us is to feel good about ourselves, this underlying agenda influences how we work. So, what should the benefit of our work be to us then?

A while back I wrote the following about my working interest:

> My passion is working with people where there is the possibility of real, healthy emotional contact, where truth is honoured, and reality takes precedence over illusions.

So, now I look at this statement and think: is this approach an exploitation of my clients? Of course, it is true that when I am a witness to 'real, healthy, emotional contact' it brings up good feelings in me - a release of oxytocin and other pleasant hormones, but is this, then, an exploitation?

I know that one of the satisfactions of doing my work is that I am always learning something new about what it is to be human, and within that, what it is to be me. At times I think of stopping working, 'retiring' and just looking after my land, my chickens and my sheep, but in the end, I have not taken that step yet. And the reason I don't take that step seems to me to be that I still enjoy the discovery, the exploration, the uncovering of more truths about us, and therefore about me, and I enjoy seeing others make these discoveries about themselves.

The revelations that come through witnessing, facilitating and being part of IoPT explorations continue to fascinate me. Witnessing contact between others feels good to me. Watching the impact of a revelation, a truth, of reality as it is on someone else, impacts me. Having good contact with others who have joined this venture of understanding ourselves through IoPT inspires me. I want to be involved in this IoPT-informed community. I want to make some contribution to the future in a way that involves me and gives me satisfaction.

What about you?

What is your answer to the question "Why do you choose to work as an IoPT practitioner?"

--------------- ⌀⌀ ---------------

Illusions of love

I don't want to give up on all the beautiful music and love songs I have listened to and loved during my life ....

One of my favourite Bob Dylan songs (and there are a lot in this category!), is "I've made up my mind to give myself to you". Yes, well, that *is* a challenge from an IoPT perspective!

Such a beautiful song, and, in some way a beautiful sentiment …
but …

Put an IoPT perspective on the title and the song; this is of course a song that evokes the Trauma of Love and the accompanying illusions of love. I can give myself to you, I relinquish myself to you, as the substitute for my mother, who I long to give myself to, and hope for her to love me and give herself to me.

The Trauma of Love means she didn't.

As I listen to this song, I wonder: do I have to give up the sentiments and emotions that these beautiful songs evoke in me? After a moment of thought I see the split in me. How do I reconcile the part of me that finds absolute joy and pleasure in these songs that so conflict with the other part of me, that part being absolutely convinced about and dedicated to IoPT?

I would say that (and this is a very rough guess) probably at least 70% of the songs we hear, and love, are about love …. Found, failed, heart-breaking, joyful, delusionary and fake, and everything in between. Ideas about love pervade everything in our lives …

Do we want our illusions of love, or do we want reality?

Was there ever really a relationship that followed what developed between Elizabeth Bennett and Mr Darcy in Jane Austin's Pride and Prejudice? We never know what happened next in their lives, how their marriage and life together was, the reality of such a seeming model for the 'right' relationship. All such novels leave us at the peak of the love relationship, and we never know what happened next. "They all lived happily ever after!" Amen!

Does immersion in the IoPT movement allow us to still be moved by such stories? Is it possible to hold on to that and honour the reality that IoPT presents us with?

How many of your favourite songs and stories are about love and the illusions of love?

"I long for a mother who loves me"

The problem is we do not long for *a* mother ... we long for *our* mother. Any old mother will not do, and, in fact is impossible. We only have one mother and the only mother we long for is the mother who homed us in her womb, birthed us, and perhaps rejected our love for her, and did not love us. And we cannot make our mother love us.

That is the reality, and that is so painful.

"I long for my mother's love"

This sentence will set you free ... but it isn't just a sentence ... it is the link to the deepest feelings of our pain of not being loved and not being wanted as a baby, and until the pain is really felt, it is just an idea, a flat sentence of minimal meaning.

Many important things can be said, but they only have real meaning when said with an openness to the feelings they connect us to.

"I love my mother!"

This also is easy to say, and for many of us it trips off our tongue with little connection to the reality of not being loved by her.

Sometimes it is said as if the idea is common: *all* children love their mother ... said in the context of the idea that all mothers love their children, which we know, in IoPT, is simply not true.

To say 'I love my mother' when deeply in touch with the reality of her lack of love for us ... that is another matter.

Can we admit this? The child part of us that still loves her, after all we have suffered at her hands, all the terrible acts of perpetration, how painful the fact that she did not want us, or love us, what the effect has been on our life, that makes it a different thing. To admit that, in spite of everything, we still love her, and long for her love of us ... yes, therein lies our pain.

It seems to me that the reason we long for her love is *because* we love her. If we didn't love her, it is unlikely that we would care if she loved us. The danger is that if we don't include this then we suffer quietly the shame of it, that we still love her despite the perpetration and lack of love from her. Then we stay with the notion that my mother is a perpetrator, and that may force us to deny this painful reality: I still love her. The paradox is not just that we long for her love, but that we actually continue to love her from the child part of ourselves despite everything.

Intention: "I am right"

This intention is a message to the mother. This is the subtle way we keep the mother there, that is why she is still there. The declaration "I am right" asks for the other, primarily the mother, to agree, to see us and acknowledge that we *are* right. We are still wanting something from someone else; recognition, agreement, validation ... love. Otherwise, this intention is meaningless ... why set it other than because I do not feel I am right?

"I love my mother, and I long for her love more than I long for love of myself." That is the solution ... then we can become the person who can say, with confidence and quietness, "Yes, I am right".

Intention in the 'name box'

Why I like to have the enquiring person's intention in their name box when working online, along with their name ...

My view is that the most important thing for the practitioner to keep in their awareness is the intention, how it is worded, what it means, the changing nature of what it means as the process continues, which words are represented and so on. When we were all working in person the intention was put up on a whiteboard, and was always there for all to see throughout the process, most importantly for the practitioner to see, and for the enquiring person to stay in touch with. That was simple.

When we moved to working online there was a question as to how to have this intention stated and where. Most people have followed Franz Ruppert's lead in this and put the intention in the 'chat'. I have not done this. Instead, I ask the person to re-name themselves, keeping their first name in their name box with a dash after that, and then put their intention. For example:

Vivian - I want my life.

I like it this way for the following reasons:

1. It is clearly and constantly visible, so anyone can see it and remind themselves of what the original stated intention was.
2. I do not want to have to call up the chat to remind myself, if I am not taking notes. Quite often in the online process a representative may feel the need to turn off their video and may only communicate through the chat. This means that if anyone, including the enquiring person, wishes to remind themselves of the intention they may have to scroll through other chats to find the intention. It just is not plainly visible.
3. I always ask the person to keep their first name in the name box to remind all of us that this person is more than their intention. Their intention is simply what they are exploring and attending to right now, but they are themselves as well, distinct from this intention.
4. The danger is that, as the enquiring person, we may collapse into the difficulty, as expressed in the intention and forget that as ourself we have the necessary resources to make this enquiry. These resources

reside in who we actually are, as expressed in our name at this moment. The intention expresses the difficulty, but this is only part of the person.

If you are a practitioner perhaps experiment to see which works better for you.

--------⚬⚬--------

IoPT and abortion rights

This was originally a blog post on my website in response to the news that the Supreme Court in the USA were about to overturn a legislative decision from 50 years previously commonly known as Roe vs Wade, which has made abortion legal in the USA since then. As IoPT practitioners the issue of survived abortion attempts is quite common in our work, and so I thought it would be helpful to open up the topic more within the IoPT community.

*

At this time, May 2022, the United States Supreme Court are about to reverse a legal decision that has been in place for more than 50 years that has allowed abortion and reproductive rights to women. If this goes through then abortion will be illegal in many states of the United States of America. In my view this is a phenomenal and retrograde event. It means that it will be illegal for a woman to abort the child of incest and rape, and possibly even if her health and life are at risk besides. In my view the choice should be one of personal conscience, not of people one has never met, will never meet, and who know nothing about you.

In fact, at this moment, it is illegal for women to terminate their[7] pregnancies in any circumstances in 24 countries, with a further 37

---

[7] Note the use of the possessive word 'their' as in "their pregnancies". It is important to recognise the issue as an issue of the woman, not the state.

countries restricting access in any situation except where the mother's life is in danger (Guardian article by Weronika Strayżyńska, 3/5/22).

I want to look at this issue from within the IoPT frame of thinking, because the issue of abortion frequently arises in our work, and in my view, we need to think carefully about our stance on this topic. It is so easy to slip into judgements and criticism of individuals, and that surely is not our job.

The failed abortion attempt

In our work as IoPT practitioners we frequently come across the issue of the person having survived a failed abortion attempt, and the resulting trauma of such a clear statement by the mother of not wanting her child, as well as the sometimes very painful physical effects of the method tried as expressed by representatives in their processes.

There are two quite obvious physically enacted statements of a mother not wanting her child: abortion attempt, the attempt or actual killing of the child, and adoption,[8] giving the child away like an object. There cannot be anything clearer than either of these, and the consequences of both of these for the child are lifelong. In the case of the failed abortion attempt, this includes having to live in the family environment as a child for many years where it is likely that every moment of the child's life is subtly tinged with the mother's feelings about the abortion attempt having failed. Or we could say, that the child in his very early infancy has thwarted his mother's will that he should not exist. Whatever the mother's feelings about this failed abortion attempt, they are all there for the child to absorb. Whether she feels guilt, shame, anger, hatred or regret, whether she takes revenge on the child, all of this is there to be absorbed by the child. In addition, he has to live with the constant experience of not having been wanted in the first exciting flush of his existence.

It is a reasonably common experience for the IoPT practitioner to come across these issues in our work, and some of the more extreme results of this level of being unwanted as a child are the very serious adult enactments of self-harm: cutting, anorexia, bulimia, suicide attempts, addictions, living unhealthy and dangerous lives, or living a 'non-life' as in chronic fatigue illnesses and other debilitating conditions, with all the accompanying misery, defeatism, despair and loneliness that this involves. I emphasise this degree of non-existence to make it clear that

---

[8] I have discussed adoption in more detail in the essay entitled Adoption, p2

surviving an abortion attempt is by no means the end of it. Such a serious statement of the child not being wanted has lifelong consequences, many of which, if not properly understood and addressed, result in never-ending emotional and physical pain.

The child's dilemma at this level of being unwanted can be stated in this way: "My mother does not want me and wishes that I had not lived. How then can I live my life, stay alive, *and* meet her wishes that I should not exist?" The only solution is a life of non-existence, non-thriving, often accompanied by such dangerous behaviours as outlined above. Franz Ruppert has said that the unwanted child does not know that he exists; his existence is so fragile that the fact of his existence has to be undermined and denied every moment of his life. This is the future of the child who survived an abortion attempt.

But does this mean that our stance must be anti-abortion? Should we take a stance at all on this issue? Is it our place to make any kind of judgement on such an issue when working with our clients?

In our work the issue that comes up is the failed attempt to abort the child, and the suffering of this attempt, and the consequential lifelong suffering I have outlined above of the relationship between the mother and child and the child's future life.

Why does an abortion attempt fail?

On thinking back over the years of my working with the IoPT process, as far as I can remember, all of the times where this issue of a failed (survived) abortion attempt came up it was an attempt by the mother to perform the abortion herself. I do not remember (and I admit my memory may be flawed because I wasn't thinking in this way before now) that any of these failed/survived abortion attempts were from proper medically performed abortions. This is an important point. Researching online I found statistics stating that the failure rate of medically performed abortions is low, something like 2% or less. This bears out my own experience that the failed abortion attempts that come up in our work are usually attempts made by the mother herself, and inevitably not done properly... hence the failure and the reported physical and emotional suffering of the child in the processes.

Perhaps it would help us as practitioners to think about this in our work, and keep track of whether the abortion attempt that comes up in our work is actually attempted by the mother or whether it is in fact a failed medical procedure. The distinction I think is important.

One of the problems with government legislation against abortion is that it will inevitably lead to a massive increase in home-attempted abortions, many of which will fail, and then result in a corresponding increase of 'abortion attempt survivors'. As IoPT practitioners into the future then, we can expect the issue of the failed abortion attempt, sadly, to become much more common in our work, particularly in those countries that legislate against abortion.

We have to remember that the abortion issue we are working with is the failed attempt, that means the person actually does survive with all the relevant consequences. As practitioners we are never working with the successful abortion, because the child is no longer alive and cannot set his own intention.[9] Additionally, since as IoPT practitioners we are always working with the psyche of the enquiring person, any representation of an aborted child in IoPT processes can only ever reflect how the enquiring person holds this child in his or her psyche. It can never show the reality of the experience of the aborted child. That information is just not accessible, it can only be surmised. In IoPT we cannot go into the realm of the possibility of connecting with the actual experience of someone who has died. That possibility is, in my view, the flawed position of Family Constellations.

So, I will now talk about the successful abortion. It succeeds, and the barely lived infant dies. This is true, and has to be acknowledged and faced.

There is much debate online about the issue as to whether the foetus feels pain (both physical and emotional) during the procedure. The likelihood is that it does, and this has to be taken into consideration. One way of thinking about this issue is that there is pain either way: there is the pain of the successful procedure, and there is the pain of growing into adulthood with the issue of not having been wanted and loved, and who is to say which is worse? It is an impossible argument. My own mother didn't abort me, and I am truly glad to be alive, but she didn't want me and that has been immensely painful over the years for me.of

---

[9] Of course, there are instances where we may work with someone who has herself deliberately aborted a child, but this is not the issue I am currently discussing.

My own experience

I had an abortion when I was in my early twenties. I did not know who the father was, and I was barely managing on the income I had. I was not very smart, and very into sex, hence not knowing who the father might have been. However, I was clear at the time that having a child then would have changed my life irrevocably; I did not want to be pregnant and I did not want the child. In fact, at that time, I saw it as ruining my life, and now, some fifty years later, I know it would not have been a good life for me or a good start for the child if I had not had the abortion. I still know it would have ruined the life I wanted to have, and that resentment would have deeply coloured my relationship with the child. One stupid mistake and my life was lost. That is how it seemed to me.

Luckily, I was able to have a proper medical abortion which was successful. One of the potential fathers was kind enough to pay for it, even though he knew that it wasn't necessarily his child, and supported me through it, and I have always felt immense gratitude to this man, even though I have not had contact with him for many, many years.

I knew at the time that I did not want the child, and although my attention was more on what I wanted than on the child, now, as an IoPT-informed person, I do not regret having done it. At that time, I would have been a terrible mother, and the child would have suffered my resentment his whole life, and I would have had to live with that too.

Not so long ago I was doing a piece of work with my own intention and the issue came up of my mother having had an abortion before she had me. The facilitator said to me "Your mother was a killer". My immediate response was: "Then so am I".

The facilitator was stating a fact, which is reasonable, but so was I, and in that moment, I actually felt the honour and respect for myself of living with this fact, rather than feeling guilty. I am not proud of my action, but I am also not prepared to be ashamed of it either.

Any woman who has had a properly performed and successful abortion has to live with the fact that they have killed another human being, their own child. Perhaps instead of vilifying the woman who chose to have an abortion, we can respect the fact that this is a terrible decision to have to make, and something she has to live with for the rest of their life.

I have had two personal intention processes where my own aborted child was brought in and represented, and in both processes there was an immediate feeling of strong, uncomplicated love between us. I know that this reflects nothing of the actual child, but only how he is held in my own psyche... but how he is in my psyche seems to be peaceful and loving, and that says something important to me about myself and my relationship with the fact of having had an abortion.

IoPT practitioners

As IoPT practitioners we deal with complicated issues all the time. It is easy in a way as a facilitator to say to a client "Your mother was a killer", just as easy as it is to say "Your mother did not want you". There may be value in stating the reality in such a way, but behind that there needs to be compassion and understanding rather than judgement, or else we are in danger of ending up judgemental and critical, yet another perpetrator in the life of our client. My view is that, simply because we are often dealing with the fallout from failed abortion attempts, does not mean that we should become 'anti-abortion'. We have to be greater than that, more generous and compassionate than that, and hold in our thinking what it means for the person to live with the fact that she felt forced to make such a decision.

I wonder how many women in our growing IoPT community feel shame and guilt about having had an abortion, and perhaps avoid talking about it for fear of this confrontation. I would not want this to become a topic we cannot be open about, and that IoPT-informed women come to feel perpetually in the wrong about. It is a matter of personal conscience and the psychological state of the person in that moment. For myself, I cannot change how I was then, and I am not sure even now that I would want to in this regard. I was who I was, but even so from my more evolved and peaceful place now, I do not think I would want to have made a different decision. I am at peace with my decision.

And to the IoPT community of men: amongst the many painful issues you have in your life, the issue of having taken the decision to kill a child in your own body, and to live with the consequences is not one of them. You may have been a party to such a decision, but it is the woman's body, her pregnancy, and her final decision to take such a step.

I am aware that when a woman makes such a decision about her own body, this may bring up a range of issues for the man involved. He may not even know about the existence of the child, and even if he does, he may be unable to have any part in the decision. This cannot be put to one side either. I am quite sure that many men would have something to say about such a situation in their life, and what the impact was. I would like to know, but since I am not a man, and I have not as yet worked with a man on such an issue I do not feel I am capable of making any other comment.

I realise that I am opening up an extremely sensitive and frequently fought over topic here... but who are we as IoPT-informed people if we cannot be open to exploring such issues? I do not wish this to be a final word on the topic... rather I hope it opens up a vibrant and energetic conversation so that we all can get on with living a good life ourselves, and are more able to support our clients to move in that direction too.

As practitioners it is not our job to judge, but to support reality and truth.

*

On Friday 24th June 2022 the United States Supreme Court went ahead and overturned Roe vs Wade, which means now that many individual states in the not-so-United States will ban and criminalise abortion, while other states will hold onto abortion as legal.

This was my comment on Facebook:

"What a paradox America is. They happily defend the right to bear arms, even though many children get killed in their schools, and they focus on making the schools safe rather than amending the laws on guns, and at the same time they decide to protect unborn, unwanted children, without thinking about what an unwanted child's life is likely to be, having to spend many years in the care of a mother who doesn't want the child, and may even hate and violently abuse the child. This is utter madness. It's the insanity of perpetrator-victim dynamics."

However, I understand that in reality it is nothing to do with abortion rights; it's to do with power and control, the primary impulses of perpetrators.

———————⌇———————

IoPT puts us right back where we belong ...

... in nature.

A friend of mine directed me to a piece on the internet about Franz Ruppert.[10] She was concerned and shocked by two things in this piece and wanted to have my view.

The piece begins with a fairly negating perspective of Franz Ruppert's published ideas on COVID-19 and the 'coronavirus pandemic', and continues on in a faintly suspicious and dismissive tone, stressing that his work is not scientifically validated nor accepted by 'The Scientific Advisory Board for Psychotherapy' (a German organisation). It gives a fair account of the basic theory, but highlights several things that obviously are highly contentious to the author. Two of these concerned my friend. These were:

- The idea that if the mother is considering abortion this can cause trauma to the unborn child, ("Traumatization can also arise before the birth if a mother is considering abortion"), and ...
- "He [Ruppert] denies the existence of unwanted pregnancies; even in the case of rape, in the case of pregnancy one can assume that there must have been 'a certain acceptance of fertilization' on the part of the woman."

The writer goes on to quote a child specialist as saying that this latter point is misogynistic and my friend added that it was sexist and oppressive, and 'the worst sort of Catholicism'.

This interaction with my friend set me thinking, and I realised two things.

IoPT, in its theory, puts us right back where we belong, as creatures of nature, controlled and influenced by the basic needs of nature: to stay alive, to find food, to keep safe and have the right environment in which to live, breathe, sleep and rear our young, and, crucially, to do whatever we have to in order to procreate and perpetuate our species as part of life and nature. All of nature's creatures, plants, insects, fish, mammals, bacteria and viruses and all other biological organisms, all are ruled by

10 https://de.wikipedia.org/wiki/Franz_Ruppert?fbclid=IwAR1e4XWFX4RY1rtxty
7bUMAmb3-mIA7kMPmmoPB2vz7yeeO465hhExsdvU

these basic needs, and no less are we. Yes, the human being is a remarkable creature within the overall canon of nature, but underneath all our extraordinary creativity, intellect and intelligence we are, still, a creature of nature with these basic needs and instincts.

As we developed as a species over the millennia, and found more and more ways of taking care of our basic needs, to the extent that many of us did not need to think too much about them anymore, we came to think of ourselves increasingly as separate from nature. Descartes famously said "I think therefore I am", which seems to encapsulate this separation, a statement of the 'enlightenment' period that celebrates thought as the pinnacle of humanity. This forgets the function of basic things like food (I eat, therefore I am), breathing (I breathe, therefore I am), feeling and emotions (I feel, therefore I am). To say "I exist" cannot be in truth a statement of the intellect. Existence is in the body, in the basic fulfilment of our existential needs. We can only really say "I exist" from an experience of our wholeness, our physical and psychological experience. Existence is embodied, and the psyche is embodied. There cannot, in health, be any separation of mind and body. Existence is the *experience* of existence.

To understand the two statements my friend challenged me on requires us to think of ourselves from this very basic biological and natural perspective, as well as from a perspective that understands the dynamics of traumatisation and the unconscious consequences of trauma.

The life of the infant from conception to birth is, for the tiny organism, a lifetime of experience, the like of which we have not considered much up until recently. We celebrate our birthday, the day we exit our mother's body and take up breathing on our own, but we do not celebrate our conception, the moment of our creation. Our birth is the result of nine months of extraordinary growth and development. There will never again in our life be a time of such rapid growth and development as in this nine-month period. In the womb we are separate and individual, *and* we are dependent and vulnerable. Our host, our mother, provides us with the environment in which we can make this most extraordinary and rapid development and growth, physically, and psychologically and emotionally. We live only so long as she lives, and we are healthy only so long as she is healthy, both physically and psychologically. Our dependence is on a body and psyche over which we have absolutely no control. We have to absorb what is there in our world, whether that is the quality of the food our mother eats, or the emotional state she is in.

Every emotional state of the human being involves the secretion of hormones. If our mother is in a stressful state, for example, her system will be flooded with cortisol.

"Cortisol, the primary stress hormone, increases sugars (glucose) in the bloodstream, enhances the brain's use of glucose and increases the availability of substances that repair tissues. *Cortisol also curbs functions that would be nonessential or harmful in a fight-or-flight situation. It alters immune system responses and suppresses the digestive system, the reproductive system and growth processes.* This complex natural alarm system also communicates with the brain regions that control mood, motivation and fear." (Mayo Clinic) [my italics]

And …

" … researchers say that the stress hormone cortisol may be one way in which the fetus [sic] is affected by the mother's anxiety during pregnancy. Usually, the placenta protects the unborn baby from the mother's cortisol, by producing an enzyme that breaks the hormone down. When the mother is very stressed, this enzyme works less well and lets her cortisol through the placenta."[11] (Imperial College, London)

The child in the womb of a stressed mother then is also likely to be flooded with these hormones. If the mother is ambivalent about being pregnant, and goes so far as to consider abortion, even attempts it, all of these events will have their own hormonal release in the mother, and thence into the child. The emotional life of the mother, in terms of the chemistry of humans, communicates to the child. If the mother considers aborting the child this, then, will have an effect on the child, through the chemicals released by the mother's psychological state.

We, in IoPT, take this one step further. We would say that in consideration of the possibility of abortion, actually killing the growing child within her, the mother has to withdraw herself emotionally from the child, make an object of the child, and that the child will sense this. Emotionally all the child wants from the mother is her love, her acceptance of him. However, this 'love' is also a chemical reaction and, if absent, the child will feel its absence. The well-known chemical of 'love' is oxytocin, and studies show a slow increase in the release of

---

[11] https://www.imperial.ac.uk/news/70181/stress-womb-last-lifetime-researchers-behind/#:~:text=Usually%20the%20placenta%20protects%20the,her %20cortisol%20through%20the%20placenta.

oxytocin during the pregnancy of a healthy (and psychologically healthy) mother, with the highest level at the onset of birth. But if the mother seriously considers ending the child's life she must withdraw and split off any love she might feel for the child. She may even come to hate the child for existing in her body. And all of this, the thought of killing, the withdrawal and suppression of any love, the emotional absence, is likely to leave the child struggling on his own for his continuing life. At such a time of utter dependence for his existence, vulnerability and helplessness how could this not be traumatic for the infant?

When working with the Intention Method, where for the most part the 'facilitator' (therapist) does not intervene or impose ideas, certainly not until close to the end of the process, this utter vulnerability in the womb of a rejecting mother is so commonly revealed that we have come to accept that the intention to abort, even if never enacted, will cause a trauma to the child. The level of emotional rejection, which may be reflected in a physical rejection, by the mother, on whom the infant is utterly dependent for his life, will result in a trauma for the child. And, even if no abortion attempt is made, and the child is born safely and grows to maturity, somewhere deep in the unconscious psyche this experience is held, timeless and vivid, and in some way, unless addressed, will influence every moment of that person's life.

It is not that the IoPT practitioner is against abortion, but we understand that there are always consequences, whether abortion takes place or not. If a child is aborted that is the end of the story for the child, but not for the mother, who has to live with her decision. If, however, the child survives an attempt, or an attempt is thought about but never actually enacted, the child even so will hold in his unconscious the, perhaps even quite brief, experience of his mother considering killing him. If a child is not wanted, there are emotional consequences for the child, even if an abortion is not achieved, as we know in IoPT theory and practice.

That is my answer to my friend's first question.

For the second question, again we have to approach this issue from a biological and evolutionary perspective, taking into account our functioning at the basic level of all species. At this level all organisms are primed from the start to stay alive and to procreate given the chance. The basic matter of the creature is driven to reproduce whatever the circumstances. The male praying mantis presumably on some level knows the danger that after copulation with the female she may well eat him, but this does not prevent him from courting her. The impulse to have sex, to mate, is one of the strongest impulses we have. This is beyond conscious thought and attitude. It's at that level that we can see that all life created is wanted. The life impulse is to continue, to grow and create more life if at all possible.

The body accepts the fertilisation, regardless of personal ideas of wanting or not wanting in the mother. We know that the female egg holds all the power in the matter of which sperm gets through and even whether any sperm get through at all. The ovum, will ruthlessly kill off the other millions of sperm after having chosen the sperm to allow through and connect with. It is the woman's body that accepts. Perhaps we could say that it is the primitive urge in the woman, coming from the ancient reptilian brain, that welcomes fertilisation, regardless of how the sperm gets into the body. This ancient brain impulse simply by-passes the intellect. It is at this level that Ruppert is thinking.

This is not misogynistic, this is nature. To say something is misogynistic or sexist is talking at the level of conscious intelligence and social attitudes, but we do not control all things that happen in our body from our conscious mind; in fact, there is likely to be more going on in our organism that is unconscious, and so, quite beyond the issue of social ideas, than we would like to admit.

Of course, on a more conscious level, a woman who conceived from rape, and continues the pregnancy to birth will naturally be inclined to have a complex and painful relationship to the child, and this will also affect the infant. To carry a child for nine months that has been created through an assault on the woman's physical body, and on her emotional being is likely to provoke confusing and charged feelings in the mother, and the child is not immune to being affected by this. The life of the mother and the life of the child are irrevocably affected. Such an event is a trauma for the mother and will be a trauma for the child. Every time the mother looks to the child she is reminded, either consciously or unconsciously, of the assault; it is always between them, usually unspoken, unaddressed and yet deeply influencing their lives and their relationship. These are severe consequences that will in many ways influence the child's ability to be with his mother, and to live his life.

As much as we attempt, by such notions as misogyny and sexism, to socialise ourselves, to get on with each other and not function at such basic levels as we may see in the animal world, where killing and surviving are deeply interwoven, we are still animals. Other creatures have no such notions as misogyny and sexism, and do not need them. We use them to attempt civility between us, and to control our 'baser' instincts. We try to better ourselves, to act with intelligence and compassion towards each other, but often this is a veneer that attempts to cover what we do not wish to see, and in addition attempts to avoid the issue of trauma, and the resulting perpetrator-victim dynamics. Societies still deny the far reach of trauma in our attitudes. Legal and policing systems, by virtue of their established principles, ignore trauma regularly. In rape and sexual abuse cases the perpetrator is more often seen as innocent and acquitted while the real victim is often horribly retraumatised by the process of attempting to get justice. We could as well ask why it is that men so often commit acts of sexual aggression. Socially we know this is intolerable, but we forget that we are also creatures of nature, and sexual aggression is rampant in nature. We like to think we are better than this, and many of us do achieve better, but many don't.

At this level of understanding we cannot think in terms of misogyny or Catholicism or sexism. We are more likely to be able to be accepting of others if we attend to our own traumas, and the prejudices and biases of our survival strategies, than if we attempt to impose such attitudes. To attempt to expunge misogyny by force or unacceptability means we are still caught in perpetrator-victim dynamics. Misogyny is the attitude of the perpetrator, the product of trauma survival, and until we understand that, we will continue to polarise ourselves into us and them, and shout "misogynist!!" at each other.

IoPT – What does it mean?

Reflections on the relationship between the psyche and the body in relation to IoPT work.

"I BODY" was someone's intention recently, and it brought to my mind some thoughts it might be useful for me to share.

Identity-oriented Psychotrauma Therapy (IoPT). These words all have specific individual meanings when we are discussing the whole (IoPT).

Identity has a specific definition in IoPT theory, and the word 'oriented' means that the word, 'psychotrauma', is oriented towards the preceeding word, 'identity'. In a nutshell we are saying that we are focusing on psychotrauma as it pertains to and impacts on our identity. The word 'psychotrauma' indicates that our primary focus is psychological trauma as opposed to physical trauma. And the final word, therapy, indicates that this is not just a theory of psychotrauma as it affects our identity, but it includes a method of working to alleviate the sufferings that such traumas have on us and our lives.

As I became more experienced in working with the method of coming into contact with oneself and one's trauma, I saw that, even though we say we are working with emotional and psychological trauma (psychotrauma), these traumas always have a major impact in the physical, the body.

The notion of splitting in the event of a trauma experience, which is a primary principle in IoPT, is not just an intellectual concept. Splitting off experiences and suppressing the accompanying emotions happens in the body. It takes energy and tensions in the muscles, tendons and ligaments that, to an extent, can never again fully relax, because to do so would allow the trauma feelings to take over and the person would be overwhelmed, unhelpfully re-traumatised. The tensions in the body are permanent as long as the need to suppress the experiences and feelings remains.

On a daily basis our trauma is continually in danger of being re-triggered, which in turn requires extra attention from our survival self to ensure that we are not swamped by the unwelcome feelings, and so on this regular basis our body tenses and cannot fully relax.

As well as this, our body is often in a continual state of arousal or re-triggered trauma, with all the accompanying hormones such as adrenalin and cortisol flooding our system.

Cortisol, the primary stress hormone, increases sugars (glucose) in the bloodstream, enhances the brain's use of glucose and increases the availability of substances that repair tissues.

Cortisol also *curbs functions that would be nonessential or detrimental in a fight-or-flight emergency situation.* In other words, the secretion of Cortisol assumes a fight or flight situation and dulls other physical functions that are deemed non-essential to the immediate fight or flight action, functions such as digestion, healthy discriminatory thinking and decision-making, and, rather crucially, our immune system. In other words, if we are in a state of constant re-triggering of our trauma, our digestion, immune system, intellectual ability and other functioning systems are permanently under threat.

Adrenaline is produced both by the adrenal glands and by a small number of neurons in the medulla oblongata (part of the brainstem). It plays an important role in the fight-or-flight response by increasing blood flow to muscles, the output of the heart, by acting on SA Node, pupil dilation response and blood sugar levels.

Both of these hormones assume a danger, and are emergency resources, and so if the system is in a more or less permanent state of re-triggered trauma, these hormones can become a permanent feature of the physiology, causing even more stress on the body. This is happening constantly as we live our lives and face a multitude of situations that are likely to re-stimulate our original dilemma of not being wanted, of being rejected and abandoned, unloved and unsafe.

Over time, if the trauma is from very young, even pre-birth, these tensions and hormonal releases in the body do not ever fully relax again. In a sense our body may end up being in a continual state of some degree of arousal and alertness to the potential of our trauma being re-triggered. Dreams and nightmares may also be the re-triggering of trauma experiences, with the accompanying physical tensions, stresses and hormonal impact, so even our sleep is disturbed, and for many people sleep can never be a state of proper physical relaxation and recuperation.

These more or less permanent physical stresses affect our skeletal structure and our posture, and over time will become increasingly physicalised as pain and other pre-diagnosable symptoms as our body struggles to deal with the endless call to arms. The constant secretion of anxiety hormones puts a stress on the organs involved, the kidneys, the heart, and the whole cardio-vascular, pulmonary and digestive systems. In an emergency situation the digestive system shuts down so that all energy can be diverted to deal with the emergency.

"Research now shows that such long-term activation of the stress system can have a hazardous, even lethal effect on the body, increasing risk of obesity, heart disease, depression, and a variety of other illnesses." (*US Dept of Health & Human Services*)[12]

In effect, since we know as IoPT practitioners that the prevalence of early trauma is extremely high, we could hypothesise that it is possible

---

[12] https://www.nichd.nih.gov/newsroom/releases/stress

that many of our common physical ailments have their roots in these childhood traumas, and setting intentions to understand our physical symptoms is likely to take us directly to these underlying issues.

For a while I began to think that we should not use the term 'psychotrauma' when talking about Identity-oriented Psychotrauma Therapy because all trauma is always in, and of, the body. We could say that the Trauma of Identity, for example, is a psychological and emotional trauma, and yet we can also see that it will have a very physical impact on the person. In the same way we could say that a car accident, or breaking a leg, for example, is a purely physical trauma, but we know this is not the case. There is a very emotional and psychological component to even the most physical traumatic event of, say, breaking a limb. It seemed to me that trauma is trauma, and to distinguish between psychological and physical trauma did not make too much sense.

In the last few years Franz Ruppert and other practitioners (myself included) have begun to think much more about the embodiment of trauma, particularly in our work with people. Interestingly this has coincided with the Covid-19 lockdowns and the necessity of beginning to explore online working. It would seem that working with the IoPT Intention Method on Zoom would even more abstract us from the physical body, since mostly what we see of group participants is their head and shoulders, and all participants for the most part remain seated.

However, this has proved not the case. In an interesting way the embodiment of trauma has become *more* visible and *more* a part of our work since we are working online. I could digress here with some thoughts on why this might be so ... people are usually in the safety of their own home; they may not feel so exposed as in a physical group and so on. Nevertheless, the reality is that the embodiment of traumatisation has certainly become much more a focus of my work, to the extent that I now realise that to suggest the person say, during a process, for example, "I exist", is only valid if one experiences this existence throughout the whole of one's body. Existence is not a concept; it is an experience, and all experience is in and of the physical, the body.

My own position now is that it is simply impossible to work with trauma and ignore the body. Trauma is in the body and is held in the body, and in this sense for me as an IoPT practitioner I am always working with the physical as well as the psychological.

So, what about this word 'psychotrauma' in the title of our work? Does it still stand up as part of the IoPT wording, or should we just use the word 'trauma'?

My final thought on this topic is that we do need to use the word psychotrauma. The reason is that the starting point of most trauma is the Trauma of Identity, of not being wanted at the very beginning of our life, immediately combined inevitably with the Trauma of Love. These are traumas of the psyche; they involve devastating emotional and psychological experiences. Yes, they have their effect on the body, but it begins in the tragedy of being unwanted and unloved, or even hated, by the one person in the world that we need, desperately, to care about us, to love us and to want us, our mother. As much as we tend not to stray into the language of the soul in IoPT, this is a life trauma of the very soul of our existence, of our psyche in the deepest sense. This is a negation of our very existence, often even before we have grown a full body; already our psyche is traumatised and our body must cope.

The process that came from this intention ("I BODY") culminated in a deep release of the long-held cry of a child in reaction to this tragedy, the release of years of tension and stress of the determined effort not to feel this immense emotional pain of having to live in an environment where one is not wanted, and that lacks the spark that fires all life: love.

"Is this it?"

Intention: "I want this life"

There is an interesting phenomenon that I have noticed over the years in my work, and that is what often happens for the child between the ages of about four to seven years old. Around the age of three and four the child has developed enough intellect to be able to ask questions, think some things through and make some sense of what is going on around him. On frequent occasions representatives in people's processes say they are somewhere between these ages and there is a thought there, an awareness of something that can be said by the representative. Often there is an accompanying image of a child sitting on a step, somewhere on his or her own, or at a degree of distance from what is going on. And this child gathers together his child's intellect, and understands something about where he is, what the circumstances are, sufficiently to make some kind of decision how to manage his existence. It is as if the age allows the child to see and understand something of his reality rather than just react, as he must, to his environment, his mother and father. This was the case in this process. The representative for 'this' found himself sitting on his own, aged about six, and the prevailing thought was "Is this it?", and then a few moments later "Is this all there is?"

That is quite a thought for a six-year-old. Imagine this child suddenly realising the reality of what he has, and has had, to contend with. Perhaps for the first time seeing his parents more for who they actually are, just a glimpse, because of course to hold onto that realisation is intensely painful and shows him his reality stretched into a seemingly endless future. In effect this realisation also has to be split off. What to do then?

Representatives, too, often talk of simple decisions made at that time, something seen of what is now required of the child in order to survive until that time, far in the future, when perhaps he will be free of it. Of course, for a child this time seems an endless time. Children cannot figure themselves in the future as away from and without their parents. They may talk about this mysterious time "when I am grown up" but in the child's reality this is an unknown quantity, and they cannot visualise a life without the parents. And so, for a brief moment, the child glimpses through the pain and confusion, the reality of his life, and perhaps, before returning to his usual managing and coping, he makes a decision, a choice ... the only kind of conscious choice or decision he can make: he solidifies his survival strategies into a semi-consciously known construction. An example might be the construction of an 'invisible friend', or a fantasied tale of redemption. Or it might be a decision of withdraw, even to stop speaking.

———————— ✧ ————————

"I want more inner space"

This was the intention.

This was my thinking about this intention:

If someone wants "more inner space", then their experience is that they do not have enough inner space, and then the question becomes "why?"

If we understand that the 'constellation' we are setting up is a representation of the person's psyche, then we can understand that the need for more inner space means that the psyche is too crowded. More space is required. And we can then think, if the psyche is "too crowded" … not enough space, what or who is it that takes up the space? And the logical answer is likely to be the 'invading mother', or at the very least the 'invading perpetrator'. The space is taken up by something that is alien, that does not really belong there.

After all, if there is a need to set an intention, it is because there is a problem the person cannot resolve on their own. They cannot stay in their healthy 'I', and this must mean that the underlying issue must involve a trauma of some kind.

This speculation was borne out by the reporting of the word 'space':

'space': "I am very young, very little … there is too much space … there is nothing there, and there is too much space. No one is there."

For me, this indicates a young child for whom there is too much space because there is no loving and contacting mother in the space for her to be in contact with. The child is in the space on her own and alone.

'space' continued, saying: " … and I feel pressure on my back"

In my view this indicates where the mother actually is, behind the child, putting pressure on the child.

This was borne out later when a representative for the mother was brought in:

'mother': "I want a well-educated child! You must be educated!"

Right from the start, then, we can understand that the presence of the mother was a pressure for the child, and that there was no possibility of contact. Real contact, perhaps the possibility of loving contact, can only happen when the mother and child face each other; the child can look into the eyes of the mother and see and feel the mother's love. This reported situation is not at all like that, but the mother is still there, in the pressure on the back. (Perhaps have a look at the beautiful picture at the end of the essay entitled "My Baby Always Wants Feeding!")

Comment on the process:

The dilemma encapsulated here is this: in order to have more space in the psyche we have to eject what is alien in the psyche, the perpetrator, the mother.

The idea that we have to eject (reject) the mother from our psyche brings us into direct contact with the underlying issue, the child's understandable and persistent longing for the love of the mother. To turn away from the mother, and towards oneself puts us in contact with the deepest pain of not being loved and not being wanted by our mother, and the only possible solution is to face it and give up on the hope and the longing for her.

More often than not we turn away from this dilemma and continue choosing our mother, leaving ourself to our fate, and finding that we do not have sufficient space in our own psyche.

The fundamental questions are:

How do I keep my mother in my psyche, and ...
Why do I keep my mother in my psyche?[13]

--------ɔⅤɔ--------

---

[13] You will find these important questions come up in other essays.

"I want to be successful"

This was the intention

"Success is defined by the ability to move from failure to failure with no loss of enthusiasm"

(Winston Churchill)

"Fail again, fail better"

(Samuel Beckett)

What does this mean? This word 'successful'? According to whom? What defines success? Is this not an 'attribute' I force on myself, perhaps because my mother forced this idea on me, that I must be successful?

Furthermore, am I supposed to be successful for her? To reflect success on her?

The most successful thing I can do in my life is discover who I am and live and be myself. The most successful thing a lion can do is to grow into the adult lion he or she is, and keep him or herself alive, healthy, fed and safe in order to produce more lions. The most successful thing a tree can do is be the tree that it is. That's all.

From this success come all other successes. If I am truly me, in touch with myself, functioning from my healthy 'I', I can see clearly what is necessary, and I have the will and ability to do what I want to do in the way that I want to do it, and therein lies success.

If you see the markers of success as money in the bank, public recognition and approbation you are on the one hand functioning within the perpetrator-victim dynamics of society's tricky perspective of what success is, and on the other hand relying on identification as validation of yourself and your existence. That is not success; that is strategies of trauma survival.

"I want to live"

This was the intention.

Immediately we can say that there is an embargo on simply living, just being alive. To say "I want to live" means that somewhere in me I cannot, or I do not, want to live. And the reason this would be the case is if my mother does not want me to live, and I am remaining loyal to her lack of support for me to live. By definition, a newly created organism, such as a child, wants to live; therefore there has to be influence from outside, which undermines this natural urge. The child is unwanted, and the impulse behind having to make such a sentence comes directly from this.

The principle of setting an intention and choosing representatives to resonate with different parts of the intention, and the notion that these then represent relevant parts of the enquiring person's psyche, means that the solution is present in the process. The intention is always true in itself, and the solution is within the representations and the enquirer himself as the process evolves. The difficulty is the person himself ... he is the one who holds the elements apart, who keeps the solution at bay, and in this sense he holds the mother-perpetrator element within himself.

The question is: Do you choose yourself, or do you choose to stay loyal to your mother and her unspoken impulse that you should not live? And every moment of non-solution in one's life revolves around this question. We cannot be truly ourselves, and at the same time stay loyal to the perpetrator, the non-wanting mother. This is a primary, and irresolvable dilemma.

To live is not an idea, a concept. It is an experience of the whole organism, the body-psyche. We cannot live just in the psyche; our living is embodied.

The solution is to *feel* alive, with all that this means. To feel the feelings, whatever they are, the emotional pain of the early traumas of not being wanted and loved. To feel the life force throughout our body. The rest is stories, distractions, thoughts and ideas ... survival strategies.

"I want to receive love"

This was the intention.

To receive love, we have to know our own loving ability. To know our own loving ability, we have to experience our loving ability, and to experience our loving ability we have to be in our body, because that's where we feel and experience such feelings. We do not feel in our intellect.

We also have to know we exist, and we can only know we exist when we feel our existence in our body and our breath; and if we feel our existence in our body and our breath, love is there anyway.

And only when we have access to our own loving ability, and direct this loving ability towards ourself … only then, when we can feel love and respect for ourselves, can we really open ourselves to receive love from another.

Otherwise, the wish to 'receive love' is a constant longing for love to come from our unloving mother. If she really loved us, we would not need to set such an intention.

"I want to stop …"

If a person sets an intention that indicates she wants to stop doing or feeling something, the IoPT facilitator needs to think, or even ask, "well … what do you want instead?" And also, to consider what might actually happen if the person stopped doing the thing she wants to stop?

To stop doing or feeling something means that there is then a gap. It is a 'negative intention'. What is to fill the gap? What do you want instead?

Underneath this 'stop' intention is the inhibition to stating a want: What does the person actually want? An intention like this indicates, perhaps, that it is too frightening to actually say, or even conceive of, what is really wanted.

In addition, commonly those behaviours that we want to stop are trauma survival behaviours, and we cannot stop our survival impulse unless we address the trauma. It is true that some kinds of behavioural therapy may help a person stop a certain behaviour, but if the underlying issue is not addressed, either the behaviour will return, or another survival behaviour will take its place. Healing is not about stopping anything; it is about understanding and coming into contact with what underlies the problem.

*

Intention: "I want to stop hurting myself"

For example, to set an intention such as this is possibly instead of saying "I want to love myself", which is too frightening to own at this moment. To say such a thing as "I want to love myself" immediately puts the person in contradiction with the mother's injunction that the person should not exist (Trauma of Identity).

A person hurts themselves as a survival strategy in order not to feel emotions, or, because their body is so numbed against the trauma that hurting themselves becomes a way of having some feeling in their body, some connection with themselves and their life force. But underneath this, the impulse to hurt oneself is not natural, and must then be seen as a trauma survival strategy that attempts to connect the person with their rejecting mother. We behave towards ourself as our mother behaved towards us. She hurts me, so I hurt myself to have some connection with her, and not to feel the emotional pain of not being loved and wanted by her, *and* in order to fulfil her wish that I should not exist. A mother who hurts her child does not want her child; that is clear, and the self-hurting is the connection ... a seriously non-loving connection.

To set an "I want to stop ..." intention immediately brings in the mother. There is nothing I need to stop doing if I am functioning from my healthy 'I' and not from my trauma splits; to have something in me that I want to stop doing immediately puts me in conflict with my mother.

———————— ✿ ————————

"I want to value myself"

This was the intention.

I want ... I *still* want my mother ... but I'm fed up with that; I want something new! I want myself.

That is all this means ... If I value myself, I have to turn away from my non-valuing mother towards myself.

Just a child, looking for love

Franz Ruppert's book entitled *I want to Live, Love and be Loved* articulates the simple desire of the newly created infant. There is a boundless innocence in this simple statement. It is not complicated and yet it formulates the essence of all a child needs and wants at the beginning of his or her life.

You were just a child, looking for love ... and in the case of early trauma there was not this real, honest, open and accepting love.

If we think about it this way, we can touch the innocence of life ... the simplicity of the child's urge to live and be. And then we can also begin to understand the omnipresent disaster for the child when these simple wants are denied because of the traumas of others, our parents.

Because of our own trauma at the hands of our traumatised parents, these simple unfulfilled wants underlie every moment of our lives. They influence our ability to live a good life, to find success in our ventures, to take care of our essential needs, to love and care for ourselves and others, and to let go of our perpetrator parents in our psyche, sometimes long after they have moved on and died themselves.

We hold them in our psyche ... this is what we see in our IoPT exploratory processes. How much we long for them to love us and support us to live, and to welcome our love for them, shows up in every process as underlying all our problems. They sit in our psyche as they were, perpetrators who, because of their own trauma, did not love us clearly and simply, did not welcome and willingly receive our own simple urge to love them, and deprived us of our innate and natural urge to live, to be and become who we really are, to live a good and productive life.

Unaddressed, this hopeless longing for our mother to be our mother and love us as she should have, accompanies us until the day we die. We do not want to shift this because to do so means we have to see the truth of her perpetration, and we dare not do that, because to do that we have to give up the hope.

To say that my mother was a perpetrator to me, while the primary key to freedom, feels instead like a sentence of death. To see her as she really was, a traumatised woman functioning towards us from her own survival strategies, feels like a betrayal of our mother of monumental proportions, and if we follow through on this 'betrayal' all hope is lost. Reality is harsh, and truth demanding.

Try saying to yourself:

"I want my mother's love."

"I am just a child longing for my mother's love and care."

See what comes up in you.

--------- ⌘ ---------

Kindness may be nice, but is it honest?

A student wrote to me after a series of somewhat difficult emails between us. We had reached a place of reasonable equanimity. It hadn't been easy for either of us. In his final email in response to one of mine, he thanked me for my kind response.

Something jerked in me. I felt uneasy, slightly nauseous and uncomfortable. I wasn't sure what it was, but I knew it had to do with the word 'kind'. My first thought was, I don't like this word 'kind' ... and my second thought was that my emailed response had no intention of being kind, but did attempt to be honest. My honesty had been interpreted as kindness. A spark of anger; I had been mis-seen. But I also realised that the interpretation of kindness was an attempt to appreciate me and what I had said.

But it still irritated me. By now, his saying of it, was of much less importance. I was more interested in why I had such a strong reaction to this word 'kind'.

I don't trust this word. I don't want to be thought of as kind. I don't trust the motivations of kindness. I prefer to be seen as honest. If my honesty is experienced as kind there is nothing I can do about that, but the interpretation of honesty as kindness makes me seem patronising and dishonest. This led me to the question: Kindness may be nice, but is it honest?

Kindness has the feel of someone doing or saying something to make another person feel good or better. Is that honest or is it patronising? Someone telling me I am kind can so easily lead to "aren't I a good person! This person thinks I am a kind person!" ... is that the first step of identification (primary survival strategy of the trauma of identity)? And then also doesn't it put the relationship out of balance? The 'kind' person is somehow better than the other, or something ....?

A person has attributed kindness to me ... what do I do with that? Do I puff up and feel good that someone else has seen me so? Or do I stay with my own view of myself, my own reality and understand that someone else may see my actions as kind, and that is their right, but my own intention was different. Somehow my feeling was that my honesty had been devalued. Kindness felt of less value, *less honest!*

But what is kindness? The dictionary definition says "the quality of being friendly, generous and considerate". But where does honesty come in this? I have to come back to this piece of writing ... just now I am lost.

*

Later: What of my honesty? The interpretation of my honesty as kindness leaves me lacking in honesty and stuck with kindness. I prefer the reality of honesty than the quality of kindness. Somehow, again, I still find I don't really trust this word kindness.

Even later: Someone else just called me kind in a conversation ... three times ... and again I felt this slight nausea and a desire to retreat from the person, and also a not knowing what to say in response. What does one say in response? "Thank you"?

But it clarified the whole thing further to me:

My attempts to live my life honestly, to live as ethically and morally as I can as an IoPT-informed person, to live up to reality as it is rather than play falsely in the world of illusions and vain hopes, all of this has been interpreted as kindness. My aspiration to live my life in as right a way as I can, which is not always easy, and I often fail, becomes slimmed down and ... well ... almost dismissed, as this super-sweet and rather nauseatingly sickly word 'kind'.

Now I have it! And now I do not need to be bothered by it further.

Letting go

Intention: "I want to let go of my father."

The only way to fully let go of someone (or something) is to really know, and feel, how much you want to hold on to them, how much you do not want to let go of them.

When you really feel the depth of this throughout your being, the emotional pain of it, then you are free.

Life does not say 'No' to itself

Intention: "How was my conception"

The representative for the word 'How' said: "No, No, No, NO!"

The Trauma of Identity is the 'No!' that the child experiences from the mother at the very start of their relationship, in the womb. The infant then, from that moment, has to say 'No!' to herself, and the consequences of this last for life unless explored and dealt with.

As an adult, unconsciously the person continues to say 'No!' to themselves in a myriad of different ways. The 'No!' of the mother transfers to the child as the only way there can be any sort of contact with the mother, and from this moment this perpetrator 'No' mother resides in the psyche of the child.

To heal this Trauma of Identity, the person has to come to be able to say 'Yes!' to themselves, and thus begins the long journey of healing. However, it is ultimately insufficient to simply say 'Yes' to oneself without a situation where one can feel the depth of the trauma of the original 'No!'. The intellectual understanding and attempt are completely inadequate to the embodied issue of the child's trauma. You cannot try to cover up this 'No' with a 'Yes' ... we are more complex than that, and deserve more than such an attempted 'cover-up' and fakery.

In this process the word 'How' was crying 'NO!' to the mother's 'No!' ... but the infant cannot act on this. It would be a despairing and desolate whisper of a 'No' to the mother, and the child cannot do this, cannot maintain this. It has to be buried deep in the unconscious.

As a practitioner, one might consider at the outset that this outburst by the representative for the word 'How' shows the mother element in this word, this representative, but you have to wait and see what happens, and then perhaps you can understand that this 'No!' is the silent cry of the child who cannot say 'No' to the mother, finally expressed by a representative in the process.

Later in this process the 'How' said that she was exhausted. This is the long-term result in the body of the continual struggle to stay alive in the face of her own internal unconscious persistent 'No' to herself, forced into her psyche from the mother.

A suggested experimental sentence in such a situation might be: "I say 'No' to myself out of love for my mother", or another suggestion might be: "I say 'No' to myself in the hope that my mother will love me". Such experimental sentences invite the person to the depth of the underlying issue.[14]

In relation to the intention stated above, we could say that right from conception there was a 'No' from the mother ... to the conception, being pregnant, having children, to her relationship with the father, and

---

[14] See the essay The Experimental Sentence, p.146

to herself. In this way there is the link into her own internal 'No' to herself, a consequence of her own Trauma of Identity with *her* mother.

Life never says 'No' to itself. The basic impulse we can see in every living thing is to live, if possible, and to stay alive for as long as possible, and that is a 'Yes' to life. It is the trauma of a mother saying 'No' to her child that the human child must suffer, and helplessly convert into an internal 'No' to herself in order to have some connection with the rejecting mother.

The journey to turn this 'No' into a 'Yes' then begins.

Listening to Jarrett[15]

For those of you who do not know his music, Keith Jarrett is a brilliant and tireless improvisor. At the height of his popularity, he would perform two to three hour concerts of completely improvised music on the piano. Generally, his music ranges from the romantic and whimsical to the ferocity of dissonance and unsettling and fractured emotions and reactions.

He is on a spiritual journey into himself. He expresses himself. That is what comes to my mind when I listen to his music or when I have been lucky enough to attend a concert, which I have done twice, once in London and once in Paris. If I think about what I am hearing in the moment I recognise the tension between the healthy 'I' pure connection and innovation, and what perhaps we could call those moments when he goes into a more survival, perhaps less present moment. The expression of this conflict emerges on occasion, most particularly for me during the more dissonant, fractured and seemingly chaotic passages.

If we consider that probably we are all traumatised, then our moment-by-moment expression of ourselves is always moving between, and expressing the tension between, our healthy 'I' and our

---

[15] If you do not know Jarrett's music, and are interested, I would suggest starting with the first movement of the Köln Concert, and move on to the Bremen-Lausanne Concerts, and then The Sunbear Concerts.

survival 'I', and then touching the trauma. Our expression of ourselves is always tinged with this continual process and movement. Then the artist, musician, painter, sculptor, is also always expressing their trauma as well as their health in every tap, stroke, splash or chip that they make. How much of the survival 'I' is in this painting, or that piece of music, and how much can we understand as healthy, and glimpse the trauma? How much is the painter's impulse to paint, to express, influenced in any moment by this conflict? What if artists and musicians understood their world from an understanding of IoPT?

If we are present at one of Jarrett's concerts we do not know where we are going ... he doesn't know where he is going. That is the nature of improvisation I suppose. Where are we going on this journey of a piece of improvised music? He is on a journey and he doesn't know how it will end, and we don't know how it will end (unless, as I have, you listen to his recorded concerts again and again!). Is there a beautiful resolution at the end, or are we left hanging on some dissonant and unfinished note? Unlike a book, you cannot skip to the last page with a piece of truly improvised music!

In his spiritual adventure Jarrett often cannot stop his own voice from adding to the mix ... not a song, but auditory expressions; he is in his music, on his journey. The audience is not there, doesn't matter, only he and his playing and his experience in that moment matters. At times he grunts and sighs, hums for a moment, oblivious of his audience.

I remember that at one of his concerts the audience were sternly told to switch off all phones and to make every effort not to cough or sneeze, or move about during the performance. The musician doesn't want to be disturbed! Some have thought this a bit excessive, but I think that this is because Jarrett has to immerse himself in himself, and any sound from the audience brings him back from that.

Living a good life

" ... if a person's psyche can develop in a healthy way, then he or she will succeed in living a good life ... in harmony with his or her fellow human beings."

(Ruppert, 2021)

"The good life is a life that questions and thinks about things; it is a life of contemplation, self-examination, and open-minded wondering. The good life is thus an inner life—the life of an inquiring and ever-expanding mind."[16]

(Journalist Gerard Hannan, writing about Socrates)

The ancient Greek philosopher, Socrates, encapsulated this idea of living a good life by stating that the unexamined life is not worth living. He maintained that the unexamined life costs you, and the price you pay is your whole life. And, more than that, there is no greater price to pay for anything, than to pay with your life. However, Socrates did not say that the 'unexamined life' was entirely worthless, leaving open the notion that even this unexamined life might have some positive value just by the virtue of being lived, of not being stopped short.

Within the thinking of IoPT we also have this idea that, in our personal explorations to resolve our life difficulties, we are moving towards 'living a good life'. This requires a persistent, lifelong openness to questioning and self-exploration in order to achieve genuine knowledge and understanding of ourselves, with a deep devotion to truth and reality, and the exposing of illusions, lies and fictions.

Socrates held that living a good life required no action that caused harm to one's own soul (psyche), and that to act to harm anyone else was also, always, an injury to oneself. The ability to harm another comes from within, the perpetrator ability within all of us who are traumatised. The momentary effect on us may make us feel strong, powerful, and less helpless, but in the end any act of perpetration towards another is always, also, a perpetration to oneself.

A good life is one that questions everything and thinks deeply about things. It is a life of self-examination, contemplation, musing and

---

[16] (Gerard Hannan on Irish Media Man website)
https://irishmediaman.wordpress.com/2012/03/28/socrates-and-the-good-life/

meditation on the reality of oneself. Thus, living a good life comes from within. What is outside of us has its impact within us, but this impact is regulated by the state of our own psyche. Our reactions to the external come always from within. We may take deep pleasure from observing a tree, but the pleasure comes not from the tree, but from our inner perception of the tree in that moment, and our wondering about, meditation on and exploration of the tree.

*

Living a good life means:

Taking ourselves and our traumatisations seriously ...

We are all traumatised ... that currently, it seems, is the nature of being human. Taking ourselves and our traumas seriously means looking within rather than outside of ourselves for solutions.

Recognising that we were innocent as a child ...

The spark of life is our beginning. Nothing before that is relevant. There are eggs in the body of our mother, and sperm in the body of our father. Our mother and father are two entirely separate beings and if they had never met, we would never have existed.

And then one egg in hundreds[17] agrees to and accepts the entry of one sperm in millions ... and this extraordinary event results in a unique creation. You.

You are a coincidence of incredible proportions. Consider for a moment the zillions of coincidences that have occurred simply for our planet to exist in the way that it does. It is 'just right' for life to have been able to form. As far as we know there is no other object in space that has achieved this, these perfect conditions for you to be able to be here, live and enjoy yourself and your life.

---

[17] "At birth, there are approximately 1 million eggs; and by the time of puberty, only about 300,000 remain. Of these, only 300 to 400 will be ovulated during a woman's reproductive lifetime. Fertility can drop as a woman ages due to decreasing number and quality of the remaining eggs."
https://my.clevelandclinic.org/health/articles/9118-female-reproductive-system
:~:text=At%20birth%2C%20there%20are%20approximately,quality%20of%20the%2
0remaining%20eggs.

And in that moment of the coming together of *this* egg, and *this* sperm something utterly miraculous has occurred: a new, completely unique and independent life form; it never existed before, and never will again.

How can this newly created being be anything other than as innocent as a new oak tree emerging from the cracked-open acorn in the earth; exactly as it needs to be in order to grow big and strong? You are who you are, and who you will become right then and there at the start of your life.

You are from the start a separate being ... separate from your mother, your host, and as such you are innocent.

However, like all newly created creatures, once you exist you are not dependent on your mother for your existence, but you are dependent on her and your father for the continuance of your existence. You are separate, and as such innocent, and you are dependent on your host. Any notions of guilt or shame, then, can only logically come from the outside. You have done nothing. You just are.

Recognising that love is innate in all of us ...

Love is chemistry. There is no getting away from it. What we term love is a conglomeration of hormones, the most celebrated of which is Oxytocin. These hormones have a primary function to support the beginning of life and the furtherance and future of life, and they originate, not in the heart, but in the brain. The prominent hormones are:

Lust: Testosterone and Oestrogen

Attraction: Dopamine, Norepinephrine and Serotonin

Attachment: Oxytocin and Vasopressin

> "Love can be distilled into three categories: lust, attraction, and attachment. Though there are overlaps and subtleties to each, each type is characterized by its own set of hormones. Testosterone and oestrogen drive lust; dopamine, norepinephrine, and serotonin create attraction; and oxytocin and vasopressin mediate attachment."

> ('Love Actually: The Science behind Lust, Attraction and Companionship', by Katherine Wu.)[18]

---

[18] https://sitn.hms.harvard.edu/flash/2017/love-actually-science-behind-lust-attraction-companionship/

We would not exist without lust and attraction, and our survival to adulthood depends on attraction and attachment. So, I feel it possible to skip ahead and say that the collective hormones that we call 'love' are in fact what life is, what allows life. There is no existence without love, and love is chemistry. Life is caused by these hormones, that then, in the innocent and pre-trauma infant in the womb, spark the necessary impulse to connect with our host, our mother.

The necessary hormones for bonding should also be activated in the mother; however it is also true that serious trauma is likely to suppress the release of some of these hormones in her. The reason for this is simple: the traumatised person's survival depends on a degree of physiological and psychological numbing so as not to feel the unbearable feelings of their trauma, and this numbing causes the suppression of these 'love' and connection hormones in the mother.

From this we can understand that the traumatised mother is not open to love in the way that the child needs, and this failure of attachment of the child with his mother, means that from this moment on, the child's life is potentially in peril; his innocence is not recognised and he has no defence against the perceptions and distortions of the parents. Any experience in the growing child of guilt and shame comes from the outside. The child is guilty because the parents see him so. The child is shameful because the parent says so, and from there the growing child experiences shame and guilt.

The innocent child has nothing to offer his host, his mother, other than his being, and his being is his love for her. All he has is these hormones of love. Love is before everything; before connection and before trauma. The child is love ... and the greatest disaster for the innocent child is a lack of love from his mother, and the rejection of his quite natural and life-impulse to love her. In this moment of the failing of a good loving attachment for the vulnerable child in the womb, his innocence is compromised, his existence is compromised, and he remains compromised and in the twilight of existence into adulthood, and cannot find the way to live a good life unless this primary issue is seen, recognised, addressed and felt.

Recognising the perpetrations against us ...

The first perpetrator the child comes into contact with is the traumatised mother. This is a truly shocking truth, and perhaps is a fundamental reason why trauma has taken such a long time to become central in our thinking about ourselves as human beings. Historically, wars and disasters may have been predominantly perpetrated by men, but men are the traumatised children of traumatised women.

If we do not recognise this reality, our ability to recognise other perpetrations against us is flawed, and our ability to recognise our own potential to perpetrate against others also fails, and we cannot extricate ourselves from the dynamics of perpetration and victimisation.

Perpetration is everywhere. Our current world functions on perpetration, on winning rather than losing, on power over vulnerability, on illusions of perpetual growth, and a visceral aversion to our helplessness, and if we do not become skilled at recognising it, and finding creative ways of avoiding falling into feeling victimised by others' acts of perpetration against us, we cannot live a good life. The reality is that, no matter how much inner work and healing we do, we have to live and function in the world as it is. Recognising this helps.

Doing the necessary intention or self-encounter exploratory work to reclaim our healthy 'I' ...

The basic work that the traumatised person has to do is see the problem and make a determined and constant commitment to himself. We have to look away from the world and its ideas of selfishness and sacrifice and look into our own eyes, determine to see ourselves, to know ourselves and to question everything we have ever thought or assumed about ourselves. We have to make ourselves central to our life. There is no other way, and right from the start, if we are traumatised, we have to understand that the fact that we are traumatised means that no one showed us as a child how to make ourselves central to ourselves. The fact of trauma means that no one saw us as important enough.

Being able to maintain a stable 'I' in situations of conflict and challenge ...

Living a good life means living predominantly from within a 'healthy I' frame. The healing of trauma by the engagement with self-encounter processes results, in time, in the strengthening and enlargement of this 'healthy I'. The traumas, as they are addressed, need less attention, and our trauma survival strategies are less needed. They are still there for those odd moments when we may get triggered. Our trauma survival strategies may show up, but we are more likely to recognise this and find a useful way to reclaim our 'healthy I' ability and step away from the moment of re-triggering. They may still be needed on occasion, but they do not rule our functioning as they did in the beginning of our journey. Living from within a 'healthy I' state means that we are more able to solve any problems we have, and we are able to maintain access to our healthy functioning even when we find ourselves in situations of conflict and challenge.

In my view it probably is sensible to see that we may never fully resolve all our traumas, but there is a massive difference from a common starting point at the beginning of our journey, where the unresolved traumas and the resulting trauma survival strategies dominate, as shown in this diagram ...

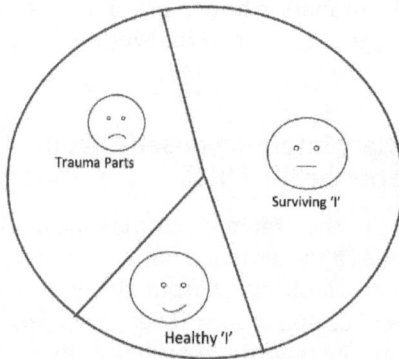

To this, where our healthy ability dominates.

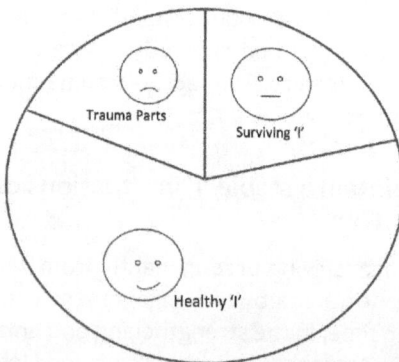

That is living a good life!

Giving up on acts of perpetration towards ourselves and others

Becoming alert to when we feel victimised, and not immediately getting entangled by lashing out and retaliating with acts of perpetration towards the perpetrator, is the functioning of a healthy I'.

If we have a consistent sense of who we really are, which is the condition of being in our 'healthy I', then we know ourselves sufficiently to see that the actions of others that aim to hurt us are, in fact, nothing to do with us at all. They come from the other person's perception of us, modified through the lens of their own trauma survival, and do not make sense in terms of what we know about ourselves, and thus can be avoided.

If we do act in a way that causes us to feel appropriate guilt and shame, then we will recognise this and make appropriate amends. Such feelings of guilt and shame are in the here and now, and for something we have done in the present moment. Our feelings of guilt are directly related to a present action, not from the confused entanglements of our past.

We are able to recognise when those we come into contact with, our friends and colleagues, may be functioning from their own survival impulses, and we will find ways of connecting to what is healthy in them with compassion and understanding, while at the same time avoiding reacting to their attempts at perpetration against us. We may also see the impossibility of living in a good way with someone and be willing and able to end a friendship or partnership that involves too many impulses of perpetration from both people.

Living in the world as it is

We have to find a way of living a good life in this world as it currently is, and this is not easy. If we really see that our human world currently functions predominantly on winning and losing, perpetration and victimisation, we can see the challenge. Living a good life is not living in isolation, and that means living in the world as it is. How can we do this?

If we are already IoPT-informed we can say:

- I do not want to do anything that harms anyone else, because this causes pain to others, and to me.
- I try not to get involved in anything that triggers unpleasant stress sensations in my body. These are a sign of the potential of perpetration from another, and/or my own impulse to anger and to harming others.
- I try to engage the healthy aspect in others ... and not their survival strategies. If I am friendly and available for good contact, I may contact the same ability in the other, and we can both avoid getting caught in survival-to-survival dangers.

I think that in Socrates' day there was not an understanding of trauma as we now have. That meant that living a good life required intelligence, vigilance and determination. The understanding that hurting another also hurts ourselves was there, but the understanding as to why there is such a strong impulse to function along perpetrator-victim dynamics, and so prolifically hurt each other, I think was not.

-------- ⌘ --------

Love of oneself comes first

Intention: "I want to let love in"

The intention implies "I want to let *my mother* in". If we want to 'let love in' it means we are looking to the external, for someone else to love us, and this implies that our mother did not love us. We look to the external for what we did not get ... we *identify* with someone else to give us love, but we miss our own loving ability for ourselves. (Survival strategy of identification).

In the process:

'Love': "I have been there from the beginning, and I am always here." [that seems a clear comment for the representative as part of the enquirer]

'I': "am I chasing love as a survival strategy?"

'Love': "You can't understand me with your mind, because

understanding is thinking. I am here ... I am already here; you just have to feel me."

Issue Holder: "Love is a Guru! I don't know if I am worthy of love!" [Distraction from the issue of connection with the representatives.]

'I': "Basically, I want 'love' to want me!" [that is the message to the mother, i.e., seeing 'Love' as the mother]

'Love': "But it's the other way round! ... you have to want me!" ['love' here is clearly not the mother, but a part of the enquirer.]

'I' to the enquiring person: "this is love ... this is all there is ... you have to get used to it."

How remarkable are the words, concepts and ideas that come from representatives in an IoPT process!

*

When we are fully in contact with ourselves, there is love, and then we can feel love for another.

In the beginning of our life there is nothing but the loving potential to be in contact with our mother. Love is the currency of life, if available from the mother, and allowed.

The greatest tragedy of our life is if we cannot receive clear love from our mother, and if she rejects our primal impulse to love her. As a newly created child our love is all we have to give her, and if our love is rejected by her, to an extent, we die.

It matters not what our mother did, or does, we love her, and we long for her to love us.

Even if we hate her, that is the replacement currency for love, and comes *only* in response to her hatred of us. If a mother hates her child for existing, that opens the door for the child to hate the mother, and to hate himself, and hate becomes the connection, and love dies.

Love is the only emotion that blossoms from within, if possible. All other emotions are in reaction to the external. We can only really love another person, our lover, our partner, our child, our friend, if we easily love ourself.

Me and my self-interest ...

... is healthy ... BUT ...

My healthy interest in taking care of my own real needs, in order to be able to be in contact and interaction with others in a healthy, respectful and realistic way, comes slap up against Society's admonition to put others' needs before mine, and not be 'selfish'!

Then I try not to be 'selfish', but this, then, becomes a never-ending burden, because, after all, there is always someone out there worse off than me, and really, I should do something to help this person ... and that child ... and those people ... and that country! In short, I should put all my efforts into helping everyone else otherwise I am seen as selfish.

Well, this is an extreme view ... but let's just say that there *is* a general pressure that says put others before yourself ... and there are rewards for that ... the 'feel good' factor ... "We all think you are great for being so helpful to others! How kind you are!" (Oh, how much I like that for a substitute identity! *I am the helpful and kind person!*)

[I remember my mother, when I was about 6, admonishing me for my excitement and eagerness to tear the wrapping paper off a present someone had just given me, instead telling me that I should take care of my friend and offer her a piece of cake. Immediately I felt ashamed of my excitement, and did as I was told ... I put my friend's want, as perceived by my mother, first. A lesson in socialisation, and another flame and spark of liveliness dampened down in me.]

At what point, I wonder, does someone say "Enough! I simply cannot give any more. I'm depleted, under-nourished, a shell of a being." This person has to stand up and say to Society "No more ... I cannot give more ... now I really need to attend to myself. Goodbye!"

And the person who cannot do that ... who cannot speak so clearly, but who, instead, just withdraws from the chaotic and overwhelming needs and wants of others, closes off and closes down, eventually, perhaps, emerging from this cave of isolation with a defiant "ME!" cry ... the cry of the truly selfish. The perpetrator's cry.

Self-care and self-interest are the themes of self-responsibility. Self-interest and self-care are healthy. If I do not care for myself, how can I really care for anyone else? All I can do is deplete myself further by putting the energy I could put into building myself up and caring for myself towards helping and caring for someone else. This injunction not to be 'selfish' becomes an overwhelming burden that in the end results in real selfishness. Because I am functioning from a depleted place in the beginning, helping others further depletes me.

Society generally interprets this focus on caring for oneself as selfishness … and misses the logic. Self-care and self-responsibility put me in a better place to expend my healthy excess energy towards caring for someone else appropriately, if truly needed. Then, caring for someone is not just another survival strategy to distract from my own needs, my own trauma.

A question here …

Why should I clean up your kitchen when mine is filthy? Or, perhaps better to say: *How* can I clean up your kitchen when mine is chaotic and a mess? What happens for me if I put all my energy into cleaning your kitchen and then I go home to the chaos and filth of mine?

Music and the body

"Rock 'n' roll. Music for the neck downwards."

Keith Richards (Rolling Stones)

Have you noticed the tremendous proliferation of an enormous variety of music during the 20th and 21st century, and even more, how much of this music puts us into our bodies?

In the main I would say that most music from pretty much the beginning of the 20th century put us in touch with our physicality, particularly perhaps from the 1950s on. Music focused on a beat, a riff, and the beat and underlying riffs and improvisations became a most important part of the innovations of music.

"Solos come and go, but a good riff lasts forever."

Keith Richards

I am not a musician and I am certainly not an authority on any type of music, but the music of my lifetime, more than anything, resonated in my body. Yes, often the lyrics were attracting, but my body responded to beats and riffs, guitar solos and singers' timings. From Swing and Jazz, through folk and rock 'n' roll, the Beatles and Rolling Stones, and all the other bands of the 60s and 70s, into the 80s, Punk, and many more that came later up until now, so much calls to our body.

I went to the Beatles Christmas Show in 1965 at the Hammersmith Odeon in London[19]. We all had seats, but no one could stay in their seats. It was impossible ... this music was not for sitting and listening to. Eventually we turned to larger venues and outdoor events so that the organisers could get a bigger audience, but also it meant that people had no real seats to sit in. It was realised that modern music, in the main, was about movement. People could move and jive and rock their bodies!

The 20th century also brought with it the ability to record music, and from there to make music from all over the world available to everyone. Native and tribal music has always been about beat and rhythm, always about the body. Perhaps we could say that this move to embodied existence has been part of an ongoing move to wholeness, and that IoPT and understanding trauma is part of it ...

Keith Richards again:

> "Sometimes I think it [music] is the only thing we've got that we can really trust."

---

[19] https://www.youtube.com/watch?v=VqwFxbllO94&ab_channel= KitsuBeatles.

"My baby always wants feeding!"

No, he doesn't!

He doesn't always want feeding. He wants you, his mother. He wants good, loving, physical contact with his mother. His mother is the only world he knows, and in the beginning, he needs and longs for physical, skin-on-skin, eye-to-eye contact with his mother. After all, the first part of his life, the nine months that was spent entirely in permanent contact with the mother's flesh inside her body ... her smell, her sound, her flesh and her touch, her taste, and all the juices and nourishment that come from her into him.

What an unbelievable shock it must be for the child, to make the most important journey of his life, down through the tight, bony fleshiness of his mother's birth canal, and out into the world, only to have all the known and familiar goo of his mother's flesh and secretions washed off him by alien hands, and put into material clothing with no direct contact with his mother's flesh?

And then, perhaps put into a cot, his own private (and loveless) cot, perhaps even in his own room ... no wonder this baby cries.

No, he doesn't want feeding; he wants his mother, her smell, her taste, her sound, her warmth and skin, her love. That is what he is crying for. He may suck and feed for a few moments, but this is just the sign ... he wants a warm, loving feeling in his body as his skin comes into contact with hers, and he sees her eyes looking for his, and sees love in her eyes, that she loves him.

"I see you seeing me"
("I [the child] see you [mother] seeing me.")
(Daniel Stern, 1934-2012)

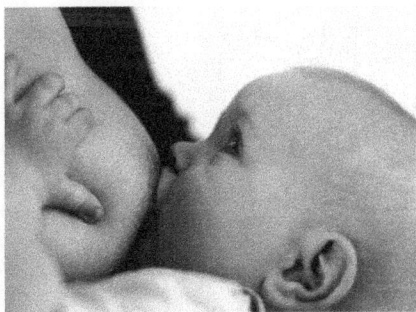

My Book

Intention: "I my book"

I did a personal process just before my last book[20] came out in order to look at what my book was to me. I had two representatives, 'I' and 'my book'. It was an individual session, so I was to do the representations, with some help, if required, from my colleague who was facilitating.

I resonated first with 'I', and immediately, and somewhat unexpectedly, felt a deep rush of love for Vivian, sitting as a marker on my desk. It was completely in my body, and reduced me to tears.

When I resonated with 'my book' I immediately felt a sense of being separate from Vivian and from 'I' ... and I didn't want the word 'my' in my name; I was just 'book'.

In the resonance as 'my book', I said to Vivian: "Now I am not yours. You must let me go and get on with something else. I am now nothing to do with you. Let me go."

I realised 'my' book is not me. It is now 'the' book, or 'that' book. I am free of it, free to just be me again. The book, like a child, has its own life and that is nothing to do with me. People may judge or assess me through their contact with my book, and I can do nothing about that, but it isn't me; that is the book. I am more than the book.

----------ᐧᜓᐧ----------

My mother broke my heart

The solution is to take your heart back from this perpetrator mother, and keep it for yourself, to love yourself.

That will mend your broken heart.

----------ᐧᜓᐧ----------

---

[20] *'Trauma and Identity'* (2021)

My mother didn't want me ...

Is that really true?

Within the IoPT-informed world we have become used to this idea, and to us it has come to be a familiar notion, even normal.

But as practitioners we have to remember how completely shocking this idea is to the wider world. As practitioners, we cannot just say to a client: "your mother didn't want you" and expect this to be received as a tolerable and easily acceptable idea. For most people this is an entirely shocking idea, and if delivered from a perspective that expects it to be easily accepted, as an IoPT therapist you are in danger of making an irreparable enemy of your client.

Hard truths need to be delivered with compassion.

———————— ༐ ————————

My mother is not the problem

The problem is how I, now as an adult, cling on to her.

Now, in the present, she is not the problem. She is just another human being, traumatised and wrapped up in her own struggles.

If I keep wanting her recognition, her love, longing for her, then I keep myself trapped in my own trauma struggles.

It is our choice.

———————— ༐ ————————

"My mother left me in a box"

Intention: "I stay in myself"

First to say, the 'box' was the kind of cage made to keep children in ... called in English a 'play pen'. But because of the translation issue it came out in English in this process as a 'box', which actually was quite appropriate.

'Stay': "My mother left me in a box! I am in the box, and I feel watched. It's like as if a nurse watches, to take care of diapers and so on. Why do you look at me in the box? Why don't you lie with me and hold me? I feel like an object being watched. I don't want to be looked at; I want to be held."

'I': "I want to stay with myself without contact with my mother!"

For the infant child this is impossible. It reflects the absolutely impossibility for the baby of existing without the mother.

'I': "She [mother] took my scream! She took everything!"

Again, this shows absolutely the impossibility for the child of holding on to herself as a baby, even holding onto her own scream.

When a representative for the mother was brought in it became clear that the mother had wanted to kill her child. The enquiring person corroborated this ... she knew that her mother had wanted to kill her, but had never said it out loud before.

Then we are in the realm of hate, and the question then becomes: How does an infant survive the hatred and desire to kill of the mother?

The answer to this question is self-hatred. Hate follows hate, and the hatred from the mother becomes the only thread of connection for the child; the child then comes to hate herself.

If you think about this for a moment: how *does* an innocent baby, perhaps experiencing this even before birth, stay alive in such a black, hating and dangerous environment? There is no alternative for the baby than to find an existence in this sea of hatred and potential violence. This hatred becomes her only anchor, and self-hatred the only solution, and thus the child's path into adulthood is set.

The tension is between the natural joyful lifeforce impulse to live, and the need for connection with the mother who does not want the child to live. The latter wins, and the lifeforce then suffers.

At the end of a process I have facilitated I am so often struck by the absolute miracle that someone could survive what they have suffered at the start of their life. Trauma survival is extraordinary.

"My therapist says ... "

This is a cliche often trotted out in books and movies, intending to be a reasonably authentic portrayal of one's relationship with one's therapist, perhaps at times slightly tongue in cheek, but nevertheless, I think, a summation of the perceived nature of psychotherapy. I have heard conventional psychotherapy colleagues of mine, same sort of age as me, still working with clients, and still seeing their own therapist fairly regularly, say exactly this phrase.

I cannot hear this without hearing it as the outsourcing of identity and authority onto the external, in IoPT language, identification. 'My therapist' becomes the source of validation, the authority of who I am, influencing the choices I make.

Identification is the primary survival strategy of the Trauma of Identity, the trauma of not being wanted by one's mother at the beginning of one's life. The trauma for the child is of finding that a connection with his mother is not simple, not available, that she doesn't see her child, nor attend to her child, in effect does not want her child for who he really might be and become.

The mother may want her child for a variety of reasons that are personal to her, but the child himself as he is, is not wanted, and only ever seen for what he can provide or do for his mother, or in many instances he simply is not seen at all in any meaningful way. The unwanted child is a nuisance to be endured, or an accessory to the mother's own lack of identity, her own Trauma of Identity. The essence of the child's own personal identity and existence is not valued, not considered, not seen, and must be split off, and the adjustment is as if this individual identity of the child never existed. Franz Ruppert has said that the unwanted child grows into an adult who, at some level, does not really know that he exists in any meaningful way. His existence is forever dependent on the parental perspective.

This is the tragedy of the unwanted child: the child's own particular individuality and being does not matter to his parents. The parents' ideas and requirements of the child prevail, and the only possibility of survival in this context for the child is to lose himself and adjust to the external, identifying with what the mother wants and sees him as and for. The child's internal reference as to who he actually is becomes lost, and the only option is to find a reference for his existence with the external, the mother's ideas, attributions, wants, and prejudices towards the child. Identity becomes identification.

Identification in everyday adult life shows in a variety of ways, but the primary underlying mode is the outsourcing of the basic authority as to who I am onto an external phenomenon, a person, group, ideology, religion etc. It doesn't matter what the external phenomenon is, whether person or institution or ideology or religion, the issue is the transference of myself from within myself to something or someone external to myself. This becomes a permanent feature of the person's life, where the authority and reference for who the person is, their continuing existence, is outside of the boundary of the person. This, of course, is the root of people's lack of self-confidence and ability to succeed in their life in the best possible way. If the person is not connected with himself, and has to have affirmation and confirmation from the external, he is always vulnerable to the vagaries and vulnerabilities of the external 'authorities'. This, then, becomes the source of immense confusion and personal vulnerability. There is no self-confidence in this, and there can be no meaningful success in his own life. Access to his own wants has been subject to a take-over, rendering him confused in his wanting, and so in any decisions about his everyday life, always looking outside of himself for solutions, decisions, validation and support.

A therapist is always in danger of becoming another external source of validation and identification. I suppose a good therapist knows this, but as I am an IoPT facilitator now, I am so far away from conventional psychotherapeutic thinking that I do not know.

Nature abhors a vacuum

Any spare patch of earth or crack in concrete, no matter how small or lacking in good soil, nature will fill it, because nature must fill the space ... every opportunity has to be taken.

The traumatised psyche, too, abhors a vacuum, perhaps because the emptiness of mind is dangerous. If we do not fill it with thought and activity, the danger is we will feel our split off trauma feelings. The mind works tirelessly and fiercely to make sure there is no quiet, no space, no void.

Perhaps this is the reason why meditation is so difficult, or even I could say, impossible. The practice of meditation is to quieten the restlessness of the mind[21], to sit in the void, the space, the emptiness, and whether the practice is focusing on a mantra, or attempting to focus as an observer on the rampant thoughts of the mind, the aim is to quieten this activity.

But if we understand trauma, we can see how impossible this is, because the activity of the mind is our survival strategy. To quieten the mind invites that which is held within the psyche, suppressed and split off, into the space, and so we fill the space with distractions and muddles, thoughts and diversions for fear of feeling our trauma emotions. So, the meditation becomes a battleground with oneself. More discipline then is required, and then meditation becomes a discipline and the split between aspiration and reality remains. The person is in a constant fight with themselves.

As we heal our trauma, our survival strategies drop away, and our mind naturally quietens. A healthy 'I' does not need the noise. Decisions are clear, choices are made, problems are solved with a clarity of thought uninterrupted by the noise of the traumatised psyche. The healthy 'I' psyche welcomes the quiet and rests in the void.

I remember, back in the 1980s when I was studying Gestalt theory in order to become a therapist, my main trainer who, while a brilliant teacher, was in fact, I now can see, severely traumatised, said that the reason meditation cannot work is that it requires letting go of the

---

[21] What the Buddhists call uddhacca-kukkucca – the inability to calm the mind and focus one's energy.

ego. "How can you possibly let go of what you do not have!" she said[22].

I don't think that a state of meditative quiet is about letting go of one's 'I'. I think it is a process of becoming more in one's healthy 'I', and less disturbed by our trauma and trauma survival strategies. The noise in our psyche, then, the 'restless mind' is the noise of trauma distraction. Heal the trauma and the 'I' can be quiet.

*

There is a Zen question by the teacher to the student: "which side of the door did you leave your shoes when you came in?" There are different versions of this question, but all Zen questions are paradoxes with the intention, as far as I can understand it, of shaking up the established form of thinking and supporting in-the-moment awareness.

The healthy 'I' knows and is conscious of what is important in this moment. Is it important and useful in this moment to remember which side of the door I left my shoes?

—————⚬⁄⚬—————

Needs and wants

Needs are about staying alive;

wants are about being alive.

---

[22] The word 'ego' is a difficult word because it has different contextual meanings. One is one's sense of self, ranging from what we might recognise as a healthy 'I' having a good and clear sense of self, to an inflated and unrealistic, even grandiose, sense of self, which we would recognise more as verging on perpetrator-survival.

In Buddhism, for example, ego is regarded as a problem to be overcome, more along the lines of what we in IoPT would term identification as a way of having a sense of oneself.

My trainer in the incident related above was definitely thinking of ego in terms of something healthy and sturdy... what we would term our healthy 'I'.

Note to my father ...

You didn't believe in me ...

So how could *I* believe in me?

It makes me very sad when I think how much my parents missed by not supporting me to be the person I really am. They missed enjoying my successes, and they missed the joy of helping me lovingly in my failures.

I hope very much that future parents will not miss these things in their children, but instead will find joy in finding out who their children really are as they develop into adults.

At least we have made a substantial move from seeing children as perpetrators of parents (early psychoanalytic 'Oedipal' thinking) to seeing that children are completely innocent, forced into survival strategies that increasingly distance them from who they really are, as they battle daily with the perpetration of adults. It's taken 100 years to make this shift.

"No thought to the winnings ... "

"No thought to the winnings ... one loves because one loves"

Vincent Van Gogh[23]

To love is to love ... but we want the return, the loved to love us back, 'the winnings'. Hence to the trauma of love. It's never enough. We want to possess and be possessed; we want the love of our mother in the bleak landscape of this lack, of her absence, of no love.

Franz's last book is entitled "I want to Live, Love and be Loved" ... It is of course entirely natural and healthy at the beginning of our life to want to be loved by our mother as an innocent, newly created infant.

---

[23] Van Gogh's letters to his brother, Theo Van Gogh.

So, this title to Franz's book is, of course, referring to this beginning of our life.

As an adult this 'want to be loved' is the problem. It keeps us entangled, and does this not take us back to the unloved moment of our non-connection with our mother ... to the never-ending longing for that which never was and never can be ... to the trauma of love?

How would it be if, from a healthy 'I', one just loved, with no thought 'to the winnings'. Would that be the signifier to healing the trauma of love? To see our mother just as a person, free of all the entanglements that so shattered our life, a woman, a traumatised woman, with her own survival strategies, her deep fears and emotional pain, another traveller on the journey of life, another frail psyche like our own? And, perhaps, to love her without the need for her to love us?

I remember the moment when I first saw a close friend in this way. I just saw her, all my past knowing forgotten, the joys and the pains of our friendship, no thought to the future - perhaps more joys or pains. I saw her figure, her face and her demeanour as if I had never really seen her before. There she was, fresh to my uncluttered eyes, strong and fragile, one of the healthiest 'I's I have known (hence our long friendship) and yet, traumatised and vulnerable too. I saw her strategies developed long ago to survive her own trauma, and the vibrancy and energy of her healthy 'I' ... and those odd moments when her healthy 'I' failed to hold on in the face of some trigger, some slight, some hurt, some sound or act of rejection. All of this was there in this moment. Our friendship, in that moment, didn't exist, because friendships develop habits, pre-emptive expectations and understandings; we live in a friendship; it gets established, we get accustomed and over time, it becomes solid, known, enjoyed and perhaps on occasion a source of irritation, envy, jealousy, even hatred. But in some way, in the comfort of the known and reasonably safe, we lose that freshness that I experienced in that moment with my friend.

I would propose that the true sign of a healed psyche is when we can really see our mother as a separate person in her own right, with no need to interfere, protect, save, serve or change, just as she is ... another being, managing her trauma with her own survival strategies, and her own healthy 'I'. An existential separation that requires nothing of her, and that we can love her for the person she is, without any need to be loved by her. No thought to the winnings.

My fondest memories of my mother are her endless willingness to play cards with me as a child, to play with me, to entertain me, to cook with me, to laugh with me, her defence of me as best she could against my father, her optimism in the face of disaster, her courage, and the warmth of her body when she held me in my own fear and disaster.

I remember one time, I must have been about 6, and we were living in the USA, and she and I were going somewhere in her beautiful silver-grey American Buick, with deep red leather upholstery, that she was so proud of, so redolent of the 1950s. We stopped at a Gulf gas station and she got me a Gulf hard candy lolly, and as we took off down the road she sang to me, with me joining in at the end of each verse:

> I'd climb the highest mountain
> If I knew that when I climbed that mountain
> I'd find you
>
> I'd swim the deepest river
> If I knew that when I swam that river
> I'd find you
>
> Without you dear my life means nothing to me
> No matter where you are
> That's where I want to be
> I'd pray to get to Heaven
> 'Cause I know that if I got to Heaven
> I'd find you
>
> Without you dear my life means nothing to me
> No matter where you are
> That's where I want to be
> I'd pay the price of sorrow
> If I only knew that some tomorrow
> I'd find you[24]

Yes, it is true that she didn't want me; my own trauma of identity and trauma of failed love has dominated my life. At times she was cruel, unavailable, unloving and distant; she had her own trauma, and her survival strategies caused me pain and fear ... but in the end what I

---

[24] Here are The Platters singing this wonderful song: https://www.youtube.com/watch?v=ZrdTm_t29yQ&ab_channel=ThePlatters-Topic

remember now, nearly 30 years after her death, is the love that was there from her own spirited healthy 'I'.

What I remember grieving most at her death was a very physical experience in my body of what it had been to be held by her, to feel her body, her breasts and her belly against mine and her arms around me. She had held me, sufficiently, in this way, that my body grieved this loss. I know I have been very fortunate to have had this ... many of the people I work with cannot say that. I grieved fully for what had actually been good for me, and perhaps in the grieving I could let go of the pain and just love her for who she actually was, with no thought to the winnings.

A final word from Vincent:

"To love ... what a business!"

(Ibid).

He never found the love he craved. The *idea* of 'no winnings' was true, but for him, and for so many of us, the reality of loving without needing to be loved was unattainable.

My mother in her car.

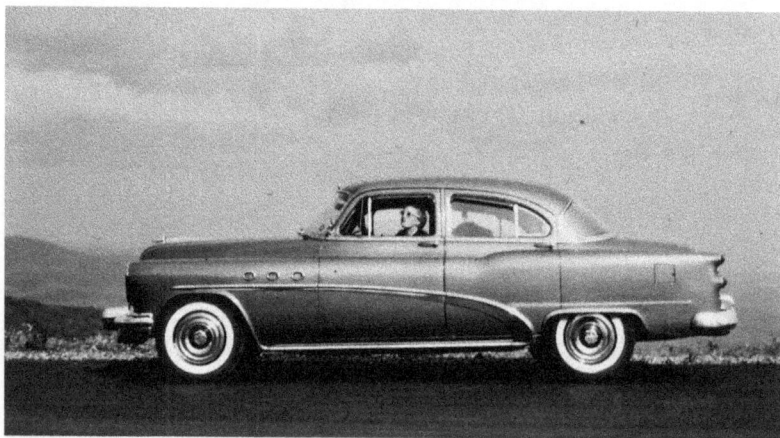

Normalising confusion

If we don't recognise confusion for what it is, we normalise it, and then we have to conform to the normalisation.

Confusion is catching, and clarity and truth within an overall normalised confusion is often experienced by others as perpetration. As a representative for a perpetrator in an IoPT process said " Truth is a weapon". So speaks the perpetrator who experiences truth and clarity as dangerous, something to be fought against.

So, to speak out against the prevailing confusion with clarity challenges the survival comfort of the confusion.

Our body cannot lie ...

The body cannot lie. It is only the mind that has the ability to imagine, to create, to dissemble, to lie. To create something that has not existed before is a form of lying; it is the creative form.

The body does its job, functions as best it can under the conditions we impose. If we do not eat well our body cannot lie to us that we are healthy. If we overindulge in alcohol or drugs, our body has to manage this. If we do not exercise this precious body, the muscles and tendons will atrophy. Our body may manage for some years to cope with our bad habits, our self-destructive impulses, because the body is the most extraordinary organism, perfectly capable of healing itself given the right circumstances.

With the terrible eating habits we humans have fallen into over the last 70 or so years, coerced, it has to be said, by commercial interests and wrong-headed advice, it is no wonder that our health systems are struggling under the weight of conditions such as obesity, diabetes, heart problems, allergies, respiratory problems, autoimmune problems, chronic fatigue and cancers. Our bodies are under siege, and politicians and industries do not help; economic success clashes fundamentally with real health.

When I was a teenager, we were suddenly told that butter was bad for us, and instead, that we should eat something entirely unnatural, manufactured by organisations that stood to make money out of the product: margarine.

We were told we should eat 'healthy' cereals, all of which were manufactured and boxed in enticing containers, and ... contained massive amounts of sugar.

Then we were told that animal fat, and even meat, was bad for us and we should lower our consumption of fat and red meat, something that humans had been eating for thousands of years.

And the food producers still contaminate our food with sugar, even though we know how poisonous it is. Did you know that even something like smoked salmon you buy in the supermarket sometimes has added sugar?

If you look through any supermarket on the planet now, the amount of processed foods (for which read packed with sugar, E-additives, salt and a myriad of other unnatural and artificial substances) far outweigh the foods of meat, fruit, vegetables, dairy products, beans, grains ... simple unadulterated foods. Processed foods make more money for the producers than unprocessed foods, which after all for the most part generate and grow without that much human intervention ... just simple care and correct growing environments ... simple earth and simple uncontaminated water.

It is the mind's interpretation of the body experience that can lie. The body cannot. The mind's interpretation is the survival strategy to enable ignorance of the body experience. That is what we have to see.

Our home is our body

Our rightful 'home' is our experienced existence, and this experience is in our body. We have to be fully in our body to experience our existence.

We do not exist in our mind. To say "I exist" without the experience of existence in our body is simply an intellectual idea, a concept. That is not experience and it is not existence.

What, then, is the state of my 'home'?

Is my home (my body), full of clutter? Aches and pains, and undiagnosed, mysterious happenings ... spots here, rashes there, backache permanently, flare ups of this and sudden appearances of that? Can I breathe properly? Do my lungs expel yellow gunk every morning when I rise from the horizontal, which has allowed the poisons to seep up from below? Does my skin itch and irritate so that I am constantly tearing at myself? Is my urine a rather unsightly dark orange and my shit hard to come by, or so unformed and floppy I cannot control it? Does my energy fail by ten in the morning, and then at night I cannot sleep? Do I have an unusual lump here, or a rather odd-looking thing there?

And my immediate environment, the extension of me ... Is my kitchen a mess and my bathroom just filthy? Is my bedroom a pile of discarded clothes, cigarette butts and empty gin bottles like Tracey Emin's Turner Prize art installation - 'My Bed'?[25] Can I get into my sitting room with its piles of books and unanswered letters and bank statements?

What is the state of my home?

My home is where my psyche lives. How can I have a healthy 'I' and live a good life if I live in filth and chaos and care nothing for my physical health and my immediate environment?

———————— ⌇ ————————

Pain happens but suffering is optional

Intention: "I want to end the suffering"

Suffering is the suppression of the pain of trauma. That's all. Then we can see that it is optional, but it does mean we have to take our traumas seriously.

---

[25] Art installation short-listed for the Turner Prize in the UK.

Panic and protection

A person set an intention on the topic of the panic she felt about moving from the city in which she had lived for many years to a small town in another part of the country. She wanted to make the move, but it also put her into a panicked state.

She set up a representative for her 'I', and one representative for each of the two places, a man for the city, and a woman for the town.

During the process she talked about a sexual assault that had taken place when she was a child by an older sibling. This was something that she had worked with before, and was not new to her. It is common for us to focus on a dramatic event that was, of course, unpleasant and traumatising, but in such a situation there is an underlying, and often overlooked, issue: the absence of appropriate parental oversight, and additionally an environment in which the potential of such sexual exploitation is ignored, unseen or even perhaps colluded with by the parents.

*

A short digression: how can such an event take place?

To put it bluntly, such an event as sexual assault within the family can only take place in a family environment that is sexually confused already, i.e., the parents themselves are sexually confused, perhaps having been sexually compromised as children themselves. Sexual trauma and confusion of the parents breeds sexual confusion in the children, which then so easily can become sexual perpetration, and further sexual trauma. Trauma happens where trauma already is.

A second issue comes from our understanding of the Traumabiography. If a child is not wanted by the mother, and so, has suffered a Trauma of Identity, it follows that the child is not loved, and subsequently there is not the required adult attention to safety and protection. The later assault would be unlikely to have taken place in an environment in which the mother loved her child, because the mother's love would have prompted her to provide the necessary protection. A mother who wants and loves her child, is so completely attuned to her, that she would know if something endangered her. She knows her child well, and any change in behaviour or mood she would notice and do something about.

The fact that the assault was by an older sibling also shows that the mother is not in tune with this child either, and one can only say, that she, herself, must be sexually confused for one of her own children to contemplate and enact sexual assault. The adult-created environment allows such an event to take place. Neither child is clearly seen and neither is adequately protected by the parents. Both children have suffered a Trauma of Identity and a Trauma of Love, and then become entangled with sexual trauma that originates with the parents.

The child cannot tell the parents

Another issue that is often ignored in such a situation is this question: if something such as this kind of assault happens to a child, how is it that the child doesn't feel able to go to the parents and tell them? This issue of the child feeling unable to tell the parents is so important, and so often overlooked. A therapy client will tell her therapist about such an incident, and will often add that she could not tell her parents. This statement is often ignored in favour of the drama of the assault, even by therapists, but it says everything one needs to know about the relationship between child and parents. If the child cannot feel confident of finding refuge for any difficulties she has in her life with her mother and father, this in itself indicates a Trauma of Identity; the child cannot trust that the parents will take care of her, listen to her, believe her, and take appropriate action, so she must keep such terrible experiences to herself.

So, we can see that underneath the act of sexual perpetration there is another perpetrator, the inattentive and unloving mother. It is too easy to focus on the drama of the assault and miss this underlying perpetration.

And even further ...

There is another issue that the IoPT facilitator needs to consider: because of the Trauma of Love the child becomes constantly entangled with her longing for, and endless attempts to gain, the mother's love. The deeper issue is the child's need, long into adulthood, to protect the mother, and not to betray the mother, in the underlying childish longing and hope that one day her mother will see her, and love her. So, it becomes potentially impossible for the person to consider the underlying perpetration of the mother; it is simply easier to stay with the drama of the assault, because to really see the mother's perpetration feels life-threatening. At all costs the child must protect the mother, and never betray her.

As an adult it may be that her notion of what she needs in order to heal this trauma of sexual assault is to confront the perpetrator, but this avoids the underlying issue of the mother's perpetration and her underlying traumas, and so, is ultimately unlikely to be helpful.

This is how we can see the whole issue from such a simple intention, and we can see the underlying workings of the Traumabiography.

And this is why I determined that the 'sexual assault' story was not the issue in this intention. It was already known and had been the topic of previous intentions. But it did indicate the underlying Traumas of Identity and Love for the reasons set out above.

*

What happened in the process?

In the process the 'town' (represented by a woman) became the 'victim mother' that the enquiring person and her 'I' were required to take care of. This was shown by the 'town' representative lying on the floor in the arms of the enquiring person and her 'I', and so the underlying issue then can be avoided: if the child must take care of the mother, it is impossible for the child to seek refuge from the mother for such things as the later assault.

What about the panic?

The panic this person feels is to do with the Trauma of Love and the Trauma of Identity, and cannot be resolved by simply focusing on the assault. The decision to move from the city to the town causes this panic because to move towards the mother, represented by the 'town' representative, puts her in touch with these earlier traumas. The issue re-triggers these deeper traumas of identity and love; the town is not just a town, it is the mother, and the city is not just a city, but is the father. Perhaps there was some safety for the person as a child from the father, and to move to the town re-triggers the person's underlying and deeper issues with the mother.

How to protect oneself as an adult?

The panic also reveals the issue of the person feeling unable to protect herself. This is because the decision to make this move triggers the underlying traumas which then causes her to split and go into her survival mode. Then she cannot stay in her healthy 'I' when confronted with this issue of moving, and in order to feel able to protect ourselves we have to be in our healthy 'I'.[26]

We cannot properly see issues of threat and take the necessary steps to protect ourselves unless we are functioning from our healthy 'I'. The moment we go into our survival mode, our trauma is triggered, we freeze and feel very young, and are inadequate to protect ourselves.

Only a healthy 'I' can protect you, and you cannot access your healthy 'I' if you are still protecting your mother from her crime of not protecting you as a child.

-------- ✿ --------

Peace, truth and lies

"For peace, you need the truth"

Franz Ruppert

Think about it ... don't just take it as a nice sound-bite.

The other way of saying this is: Lies produce conflict. One person lies to another, and because they know they have lied, they expect lies back, then the encounter is set: it is based on lies and can only exist as a fake relationship in which there can be no trust.

Lies create mistrust, and mistrust is the start of betrayal, and betrayal is painful. The realisation of betrayal is a shock, particularly if the betrayal is by someone we love and trust. The greater the love and trust, the greater the betrayal.

---

[26] It might be helpful for the IoPT practitioner to read the chapter in my book *Trauma and Identity* entitled 'Starting Principles'. (*Trauma and Identity*, 2021)

To lie to someone treats them as an object, not as a subject. If we respect and love someone, do they not deserve the truth from us? Always?

A mother lies to her child. What does that say about how she sees her relationship with her child? Perhaps she thinks that she protects her child with her lie, but does she? Or is each little lie the escalation of a dishonest relationship? It's not that a parent should tell their child everything, but if a child asks, should we not honour the asking child with the truth? With love? The truth may be hard, but it doesn't have to be brutal. Delivery is the key ... how we say the truth, what we say, how much we include ourself in the saying of a difficult truth, how much love is in the saying.

A teenager asks his mother "did you want me when you had me?" Why does the child ask? Where has the question come from? How is it that the thought of not being wanted entered the psyche of the child? What is the state of the child's psyche that this question needed to be asked? Does this not immediately present the notion of doubt in the child's mind? Already the question is there in the child; does this not tell us that there is a valid topic here to be considered?

What, then, does the mother or father answer? Can the mother admit the truth to herself, or does she live a lie? Has she banished from her psyche the truth in order to be able to commit herself to bringing up the child? What is the truth, and can she treat her child with the honour and honesty he deserves?

A mother answers "Of course I wanted you!" Does this pacify the question in the child? No, of course not. If there is doubt in the child's mind does this answer expel this idea? I doubt it. Instead, I think it splits the child further: one part wants the mother's answer to be the truth, attempts to bury the doubt, and accepts the mother's answer, and loves the mother. The other part is faced with a dilemma: if the mother is lying what does that mean about the child's place in relation to the mother? If the child accepts the mother's answer a kind of peace may prevail, for a while. But the other part has to contend with the doubt, not just about her answer, but about her.

As much as children at the beginning of their life are primed to love their mother, they are also primed to trust their parents. The greatest trust is that trust by the child of the parents. In the beginning we have no choice. Our parents are our world and we have no option but to trust them, and to trust what they tell us about themselves and about us. We just trust. They are our parents.

We have no recoverable conceptual memory before the age of three or so, and we have then to rely on our parents for what they can tell us about that early part of our life. Even after that, we have no choice but to agree to all the attributions served to us by our parents. They, as the adults, are the arbiters of truth for us as children.

I remember as a young child being told that I must always tell the truth, and that things would be okay if I was always truthful … and then I told a truth, and it wasn't okay. I got punished anyway, even though I told the truth.

What is a child to make of that? I remember a moment after that when I realised that my parents didn't really want the truth; they wanted what they wanted, and so I adjusted myself from then on, and pretty soon I got used to lying. I got pretty good at it, and lied my way out of many difficult situations, every time, I realise now, treating the person I lied to as an object. And treating myself as an object.

Lying is a survival strategy to avoid the uncomfortable feelings that the truth may cause.

A truth may be difficult, it may be painful in the moment, but if it clearly comes from a place of love and respect, from the healthy 'I' in the sayer, in an attempt to engage the healthy 'I' in the other, it helps to keep the relationship in the realm of honesty and peace.

Politeness vs genuineness

It's not about being polite, it's about being genuine.

There was a question from two new-to-IoPT participants, as to how they should respond to their representatives when they came to do their first enquiry process; whether they should acknowledge what their representatives might offer by saying something like "I hear you" or "thank you". They wanted to know the correct etiquette of IoPT; they wanted to be polite and get it right.

My response was "It's not about being polite, it's about being genuine."

This made me think about how much of our general interactions are judged as to whether they are polite, rather than as to whether they are genuine.

Power

Power is an addiction, just as dangerous and addictive as heroin or crack cocaine.

Anyone who desires, or is drawn to gain, power over others in any way, is traumatised, and lives out their own underlying experience of vulnerability and helplessness by causing these experiences in others. They live in permanent fear of exposure and, over time, strengthen their survival strategies so much that any real sense of themselves is constantly overlaid with survival strategies. The impulse to gain power over another is the desire and action of perpetration.

Think about how much our global society and functioning is based on power over others.

A position of power in a community, institution or government is a position of authority over some particular aspect of that community, and a person who takes on such a position is not necessarily looking for power over other people. In the best intentions, he or she perhaps is really looking to do something helpful and contribute something to the community, but a problem arises if the person is traumatised, in that this power can so easily be abused and become an outlet for the perpetrator needs of the person.

Whoever we are, if trauma lies deep within us, a position of authority can so easily become an outlet for the perpetrator in us. Power is seductive. It is the antidote to the inner fear of helplessness and vulnerability, and as such it is a drug that so easily becomes an addiction. Even as heroin and other hard drug addiction is a social issue, power addiction is much more so, much more subversive, much more prevalent, and what makes it much more dangerous is that it is socially acceptable.

Fear is the weapon of power. Also, shaming, guilt tripping and humiliation.

Money is a signifier, along with public status and fame.

I do not trust anyone who wants and acts to gain power of any kind over anyone else, and that includes therapists and IoPT facilitators.

I do not trust myself when I find that I am trying to gain power over someone else. I must, then, be functioning from my survival 'I', the perpetrator in me.

--------⌒◦⌒--------

Protecting ourselves from the truth

When we say that we protected our mother as a child, it is not true. But we protect her now if we do not acknowledge the truth about what happened to us as a child, her perpetration and exploitation of us.

When we were a baby, our mother may have used us to protect herself from her own trauma feelings, from the father, from the terrible reality of her own life. But the young child cannot make such a decision, to protect his or her mother; he is too helpless and vulnerable, and must instead conform to her ideas, wants and psychological constructions. The baby and child just needs her, contact with her, in the hope that she might see him and love him, and if the mother uses the child as a protection, the child cannot do anything else but enact what the mother desires.

For a person to say that, when they were a baby, they tried to protect their mother, as if this was a choice they could make, helps the adult person avoid the truth of the mother's exploitation of them, thus absolving the mother of responsibility for her acts of perpetration. It also allows the person not to connect with just how vulnerable he or she was then. It is hard for us as adults to really understand just how vulnerable we were as a baby.[27]

---

[27] I tell my IoPT students, whenever they have the opportunity to see a very newly born baby, perhaps their own or someone else's, to look closely to see just how vulnerable and helpless this baby is.
This is how we all were at that age. We forget this in our adulthood.

On the other hand, when we are adults and we do not allow ourselves to acknowledge and speak the truth of what happened to us and how our mother traumatised us, how she used us, then we *are* protecting her, we *are* making a choice. We protect her in order to avoid the reality of her crimes, her perpetration, and to protect ourselves from seeing the truth, because when we really see the reality of our relationship with our mother, we have to give up the delusionary idea that one day, some time, she will love us as she should have done when we were young.

For the adult, who has the ability to make proper choices, to choose to continue to protect his idea of his mother perpetuates the hope and longing that she will come to love him, or even does in reality love him if he can just find the key to unlock this love. Then he remains entangled.

It is for the adult to make the choice to see reality as it is and give up protecting his mother, and instead turn his own loving and protecting ability towards himself. Thus, rather than squandering this love on someone who has spent a lifetime spurning him and his love, the person makes a different choice. Perhaps in the beginning it feels like an unbearable betrayal of your mother, but it isn't ... it is the beginning of not betraying yourself.

It doesn't matter who she is or what she did, if we continue to protect our image of her and do not confront the reality, our longing and love for her is still there, and quietly rules our life.

Questions?

"You have to let the silence suck out the truth"

Bob Woodward, Journalist, The Washington Post

If, as an IoPT facilitator, you ask the enquiring person a question, be aware that by doing so you are drawing the contact to you and the enquiring person, and away from the enquiring person and her representatives and the process.

Our job, in the main, is to support contact between the enquiring person and her representatives, the different parts of herself, not to act in a way that draws the contact into a conventional psychotherapy form that is based on the dialogue between therapist/facilitator and client.

I suggest you ask a question only if there is some information that you think you need ... for example, "Who was in your immediate family?", or "Do you know why your parents divorced?", or "Do you know how your birth was?" And even then, only if you think it absolutely necessary to have this information.

More 'psychotherapy-style' questions, such as "How do you feel?", or "What is happening for you?", draw the contact impulse towards you and away from the process. In addition, in order to answer a question, even one like "How do you feel?", actually draws the person away from their feelings into their intellect in order to form an answer. If you are really watching the person, you will know how they are feeling. Then you, as the IoPT facilitator, have interrupted the contact between the enquirer and herself and her representatives.

Sit with the silence and let it "suck out the truth".

Be careful of questions.

Real or survival emotions?

Real emotions connect.

Survival emotions disconnect.

Real emotions generate an empathic resonant response in others present.

Those present feel the emotion being expressed in their own body, and are drawn towards the person expressing and feeling genuine emotions.

Survival emotions generate disinterest and distance, and disconnection from others.

Those present are not affected by the survival emotional expression and feel nothing, except perhaps boredom and disinterest, and an impulse to move away.

Real emotions originate deep in the body, in the belly and the solar plexus. There may be some tears accompanying real motions, and there may not, but there will be some expression of some kind that comes from the deep.

Tears are not necessarily the indication of deep feelings, because survival emotions are often full of never-ending tears. There may be lots of tears and snot, but if the feelings bounce along the surface rather than reaching deep into the person, they mean little. They are a distraction.

Real emotions touch the deepest part of us, our trauma emotional pain, and those present feel that and are put in touch with their own deepest part of themselves.

Survival emotions distract from these deep feelings, and only create disconnection and distance.

Survival emotions prompt all the 'Ds': Dissociation, Distraction, Disconnection, Disinterest, Distance.

Rights of the representatives

The representative in the IoPT process is contributing something of immense value to the process, and deserves to be seen in this way. The IoPT practitioner cannot do her job without the contribution of those willing to act as representatives in others' enquiry processes, and this means that the practitioner has a degree of responsibility towards the representatives, and representatives have a right to be treated respectfully by the IoPT practitioner in their role at all times.

The invitation

The request by the enquiring person of someone in the group to take up a representation for them in their process is, first and foremost, an invitation. And as such this invitation must wait for acceptance, and not be assumed to be accepted. Likewise, the person invited needs to know that it is an invitation, a serious one, and they have the right to accept or decline.

Invitation accepted

Once the invitation is accepted the representative proceeds to do their job of sharing what they can with the enquiring person ... and whoever they are, they are always doing their best. It is true that sometimes people new to the work may struggle in the beginning, and have concerns about what they are sharing and whether what they experience is their own material or really to do with the process. However, whatever the representative says, however experienced or inexperienced they are, the facilitator needs to show respect for the person's ability as it is now. After all, the enquiring person has chosen this person, and there is meaning in that.

As an aside ... I think it is always interesting for the facilitator to consider why an enquiring person may choose someone they know is completely new to the work. There is nothing wrong with this of course, but it is even so worth the facilitator's moment of consideration. Perhaps there is something in the unconscious of the enquiring person ... something that draws her to this person, or perhaps it is a 'survival check'. What I mean by that is that unconsciously we are all likely to put in something to keep things manageable and safe. A person new to acting as a representative may be chosen as such a 'survival check'.

The process

In my view the facilitator has as much of a duty to the representatives, in terms of how she behaves towards everyone, as she does to the enquiring person. She cannot reach a useful conclusion as to the outcome of the work without these representing people, and they have every right to expect to be held well, heard and valued for their function by the facilitator.

*

Perhaps to illustrate what I am talking about I will tell you a personal experience of mine as a representative.

My experience

I was asked to represent the enquirer's mother, in an online event, and I agreed. That is the first point: I *agreed* to take up this job on behalf of the enquiring person, as a representative.

However as soon as I was brought in, I was immediately attacked verbally by two of representatives, who overruled the enquiring person's right to hear what the *representative* for the mother had to say. To be clear, I am making a distinction between the *representative* for the mother, and the mother herself. The attack was against the mother as if the representative was the actual mother.

After a few minutes of this I simply turned off my video. I felt shocked and upset, and re-triggered into my own trauma of not being valued, heard and acknowledged, and also angry that I could not fulfil my job of communicating, if asked, my experience to the enquiring person. It's not that I think that if a representative for the mother is brought in, she should always be asked to say something; it is often simply useful to see a representative for the mother, and not necessarily hear anything from her. It is that I felt completely unvalued in my willingness to function as a representative.

My argument was not with the two representatives who attacked me - after all they were just doing their job as representatives themselves - my argument (afterwards of course) was with the facilitator, who did nothing in the moment, either on my behalf nor on behalf of the enquiring person who had a right to hear from me if she so chose.

I felt unsupported in my job as a representative by the facilitator, who, in my view, did not hold the process sufficiently on behalf of the enquiring person and her right to be in charge of her own process, or on my behalf as a willing representative. (I did talk with the facilitator after the event and my issue was heard and understood. I am merely using this experience to help us all improve our facilitation skills.)

*

Representatives as useful sources of feedback to the practitioner

When I am supervising student practitioners, and we have the contract to discuss the work to some degree after it is finished, I will often ask those who represented, once out of role, to give feedback to the facilitator as to their experience of being a representative in the process. This is referring to the person's own experience while functioning as a representative. I think this is invaluable feedback for the practitioner; the representatives always have the right to be treated with respect while doing this crucial job, and they can give sometimes incredibly helpful feedback to the practitioner.

———— ᴄᴧᴐ ————

Shouting

"Those that fight don't listen, and those that listen don't fight"
Fritz Perls

If we are really in touch with ourselves, we do not need to shout.

People shout when they do not feel heard, and if they do not feel heard, they do not listen to themselves, they are not in touch with themselves.

They need someone else to hear them, because no one listened when they were a child ... and there we have the Trauma of Identity.

The need to shout is a symptom of the Trauma of Identity.

Symptoms have a history

Intention: "Why I have eczema?"

Symptoms are the survival strategy ... but they also hold the trauma.

My first thought on seeing this intention was that this exploration is about a symptom, and since symptoms are always a symptom of something, the question then becomes: What is this symptom pointing to?

> "A finger pointing at the moon is not the moon. The finger is needed to know where to look for the moon, but if you mistake the finger for the moon itself, you will never know the real moon."
> (Thich Nhat Hanh)

Every manifestation, whether physical, emotional, psychological or behavioural is a symptom. As much as eczema or cancer are actually symptoms, so too are depression and other psychological diagnoses. As much as a lack of confidence is a symptom, so too is the inability to maintain a successful relationship. Even to say that I have a problem that I cannot resolve is, itself, a symptom of trauma.

The correct question is: What does this particular symptom point to? What is the underlying cause? The manifestation of our problems is just that, evidence of something else. There is always a cause, a history of the development of a symptom.

One reason to work with the symptom is in order to suspend judgement as to the cause, acknowledging that we do not actually know. However, it is interesting to me how much our conventional thinking, whether psychotherapeutic or medical, stops at the symptom, as if the symptom did not have a history, and then attempts to treat the symptom without any understanding of why the symptom has appeared now. Something like cancer, or eczema, does not just randomly appear; each has a history of development that will cover many years, even to the beginning of the person's life. Much of this time the symptom might have been so subtle as to be successfully ignored. To focus on the symptom and ignore the underlying causal history must, in the end, fail. Perhaps with some treatment, a medical condition may disappear, but if the underlying causal history is not addressed it would seem obvious that something else will take its place, another physical or psychological, or behavioural problem will emerge.

The symptom is the survival strategy; it is the body-mind's way of managing the stress of something else. In IoPT we would say that that 'something else' is most likely to be early trauma, and in that way, we can say that the symptom is also holding the trauma. The symptom is the survival strategy, but it also holds/points to the trauma.

Trauma

Trauma is a moment of complete and utter helplessness and overwhelm. There is nothing the trauma victim can do in the moment of the trauma except dissociate from the current reality – perhaps even with an experience of leaving one's body - and split off the unbearable experience and feelings. That is the only way we can survive such a life-threatening and life-defying moment. It is a massive shock to the body-mind-system, a contraction of the senses, and of the physical structures of the body in the attempt to withdraw from the experience. The person cannot in fact leave their body, that would be death, but the experience is of a withdrawing of the senses from the body in order to survive. The physical and emotional tensions involved in this experience, and in the only possible solution, splitting, mean that the psyche and the physical can never truly relax again. At some level the entire system is constantly under a degree of tension and stress from this moment on; proper, healthy relaxation is not possible. Nightmares, for example, show that the psyche cannot relax in its efforts to complete the trauma experience. The nightmares are symptoms of the psyche and the body's inability to resolve the trauma.

The subsequent adjustment that is required, often by the infant, even in the womb, is not just a psychological adjustment, or a behavioural one, but a permanent psycho-physical adaptation in order to protect the person from a re-traumatisation ... a re-living of the actual moment of the trauma. This actual moment, together with all the attendant unexpressed frozen-in-time emotional and physiological tension, stays, split off, exactly as it was at the moment of the trauma. The person's life from that moment is one of permanent underlying stress. The 'splitting off' itself and the suppression of feelings requires permanent physical tension.

Over the years this will eventually manifest in a huge variety of symptoms:

- **Physical distortions,** for example backache, uneven physiology, the pain of which takes one to the chiropractor or osteopath;
- **Emotional distortions,** for example any of the psychological or 'mental disorders'[28] that take people to a psychiatrist, psychotherapist or counsellor;
- **Behavioural distortions,** such as obsessive and compulsive behaviours, eating disorders (anorexia, bulimia etc), self-harming lifestyle;
- **Addictions** to anything from drugs and alcohol to computer games and shopping;
- **Chronic physical illnesses,** from eczema through to illnesses such as CFS[29], diabetes and cancer.

All of these ailments have a history, and this is not just a history of, for example as in diabetes, bad eating. To really understand the history of an ailment, we have to ask the question: "Why is it that this person has been eating unhealthily/smoking/overworking/harming themselves all this time?" This is the correct question to ask when confronted with a symptom.

The IoPT session when working with symptoms

What we see in the IoPT session, often immediately in the representatives' experiences of being very young or even in the womb, is that all symptoms are symptoms of trauma, and usually the symptom of the Trauma of Identity, the earliest trauma we experience. When the IoPT process produces even just one representative that feels young, or describes experiences that we could attribute to and understand as being in the womb, we know that the topic expressed in the intention, and the symptom mentioned, are connected to the very earliest time of life. The memory of the moment of trauma, and the resulting contractions and physical re-organisation and adjustments in the body to manage the onslaught, is there. The symptom speaks this memory.

---

[28] As described in every category in the DSM V.
[29] Chronic Fatigue Syndrome

Watch carefully what happens to the 'symptom word' representative in the process, because the 'symptom' representative's reactions and changes will also be symptoms of the changing dynamics of the process.

Taking yourself seriously ...

If you do not take yourself seriously now, then all your past struggles were for nothing, and your current struggles will continue, and even get worse.

The problem is that we are unlikely to have any kind of model for taking ourselves seriously, because the traumatised cannot do this without addressing their trauma. And if we are the child of traumatised parents, they did not take themselves seriously and then as a child we were not taken seriously by them.

Additionally, society does not take us seriously. We end up with no model for how to take ourselves seriously, and no support for it. We do not matter to anyone, and we do not know how to matter to ourselves.

Taking yourself seriously means taking the fact that you are traumatised seriously. And taking the fact that you are traumatised seriously means doing something about it. Nothing else will do, and no one else can do this for you, not your partner, your child, your friend or your therapist.

And the IoPT practitioner cannot do this for you either, but she can show you ways to heal yourself and your trauma, if you take it seriously.

Tasting cheese

"Information is not necessarily the truth"

Yuval Noah Harari

Intention: "I want to know"

What is knowing?

Knowing is about feeling. We can 'know' facts or information that we are told, and that may help us to navigate our life, but real knowing involves feeling and experiencing, otherwise it is just 'facts' or information we have been told, and information is not necessarily the truth.

We cannot know cheese if we do not taste it; tasting is sensing, feeling and experiencing. When we taste a cheese, then perhaps we can say we know this cheese, but no one else can tell us what cheese really tastes like, the taste and after-taste, the texture, the smell, the feel of it in our mouth.

If we want to *know* ourselves, we have to be available to feel what is in our body, and that, of course, is where the trauma feelings are held.

———— ⌀ ————

Teenage rebellion

We hear a lot about teenage rebellion, but what exactly is it? What is the teenager rebelling against? How can we think about teenage behaviour from an IoPT perspective.

Here is something about this topic from Wikipedia:

Teenage rebellion is a part of human development in adolescents in order for them to develop an identity independent from their parents or family and a capacity for independent decision-making. They may experiment with different roles, behaviors, and ideologies as part of this process of developing an identity.

Teenage rebellion has been recognized within psychology as a set of behavioral traits that supersede class, culture, or race ... the child's allegiance to parental authority and worldviews can weaken after the discovery that parents, like themselves and everyone else, are mortal.

This realization creates an unconscious need for security that is broader than what the parents alone provide. This can lead to new cultural allegiances, in the search for a more enduring sense of meaning. Teenagers seek to perceive themselves a valued contributor to aspects of culture that more convincingly outlive or transcend the mortal individual's lifespan. However, since the parents also instil their cultural beliefs onto the child, if the child does not come to associate their parents' mortality with their cultural beliefs, the chances of rebellion decrease.

You can see from this piece how the general idea of teenage rebellion is the need to "develop an identity". The IoPT perspective would understand this, but only because the real identity of the child was lost so much earlier in the child's life, as the Trauma of Identity.

So, from this perspective, the child tries to find an 'identity' as a teenager to substitute for this very early loss, and the 'identity' discussed in the Wikipedia piece is, in IoPT terms, an impulse to find some other identification (the primary survival strategy of the Trauma of Identity), a substitute for their earlier survival identification with the needs, wants, ideas and attributions imposed by the parents. But this is still identification, and not the basis for a true identity.

IoPT's definition of identity is:

- All of who I am within the physical and psychological boundary of myself ...
- Including what is conscious and what is unconscious;
- Including all my experiences, good or bad, known or unknown, denied or allowed;
- Including all my splits and my traumas, even from my time within the womb.

And further:

- If I deny any of this, I am no longer fully in my identity ...
- I am split between what I allow and what I deny.

And finally:

- My identity becomes real to me through feeling it, through allowing myself to feel in my body my experiences, both immediately in the here-and-now, and those experiences that have been frozen in time and split off in the trauma survival process.

So, the conventional perspective on identity, as described in the Wikipedia piece, is something that is found outside of us and something that we can develop, rather than who we actually are in terms of IoPT thinking.

The Trauma of Identity splits us from ourselves, from our real identity, and then we look for an 'identity' outside of ourselves. That is identification, and can only ever be a substitute.

The "discovery that parents ... are mortal"

The general idea in the Wikipedia piece is that as the child grows to teenage-hood there is the growing awareness of the parents' vulnerability and failings. This quote is followed by: "This realization creates an unconscious need for security that is broader than what the parents alone provide."

The IoPT version would say that, if there has been a Trauma of Identity, there definitely was not any proper security for the child, and so the search for this is then extended to the more external world ... further identifications.

An IoPT understanding of teenage rebellion ...

But enough of this! How would we think about this phenomenon of 'teenage rebellion' within the IoPT perspective?

My own idea is that, with the development of teenagers' intellect and ability to think about themselves and their life, there is a need to expose the lies and falsehoods perpetrated on them by the parents. Another way of understanding this is to say that the teenager starts to see through the parents, and challenge their lies and dishonesty ... their inauthenticity ... in effect, their survival strategies.

So, to put it more simply we could say that teenage rebellion is the child's rebellion against the survival strategies of the parents.

But the teenager is caught between his or her natural desire for the truth and authenticity, his emerging intellectual realisations, and the still-existing underlying child-longing for his parents to be right, to be trustworthy, the parents they should have been, and to love and see him. The 'empress' mother has shed her clothes ... some reality and truthfulness comes through; it is perhaps a relief, but it is also devastating. The teenager goes out into the world, and finds a degree of truth, but the whole truth is intolerable.

And so, the teenager rebels ... and then goes home.

Telling the stories keeps you stuck

"Let me question always and doubt deeply – especially my own motives."

Jiddu Krishnamurti[30]

The primary purpose of any kind of exploration is to find something that you didn't know before, and the stories that we have about our life cover over the painful realities that we avoid.

There are two kinds of stories that deflect us from reality and truth: the stories we are told by others, primarily our parents and family and our educators, and the stories we make up for ourselves in order to manage the reality of our childhood.

Either way these stories are a construction, but they are not the truth, and while they may help us survive our childhood, if we really want to know who we are we have to question everything. If we keep telling and living by the stories, we protect ourselves from looking into the truth of who we are.

---

[30] In J. Krishnamurti. The Years of Fulfilment (A Biography of J Krishnamurti by Mary Lutyens Book 2)

You are not the stories others have told you, nor are you the stories you may have constructed to help you survive. These are just stories, and the veracity of all of these stories should be up for exploration and questioning, always.

Terror and the war within

My own process

Intention: "I - Putin - Ukraine"

I set this intention during the invasion of Ukraine by President Putin. I thought before the start that the representative for Putin would probably be my father, and the representative for Ukraine might have some resonance with my mother.

Quite soon in the process it was clear that the reference was to the war between my parents, and my vulnerability as a child in this. The representative for Putin did indeed become clearly my father, and the representative for Ukraine also became similar to my mother. 'Putin' was aggressive and accusing and 'Ukraine' meanwhile virtually fell asleep. This reflected the aggressive nature of my father, and how my mother dealt with his aggression. I, as a child, was caught in between their war and abandoned by my mother to the aggression and intolerance of my father.

My 'I' felt very young and vulnerable, and unsupported by me, and eventually turned off her video, and I was alone with my parents, just as I had been as a child.

As the process progressed 'Putin' became more aggressive towards me, and said that I was not being real, I was not being honest. This struck deep within me, as I value my ability to be real and to be honest ... this was shocking for me, and I felt very attacked and vulnerable, to the extent that I felt the need of my facilitator. I felt no support from anyone in the process. 'Ukraine' was virtually absent, 'Putin' I experienced as attacking and accusing, and my 'I' was a very vulnerable child that I felt entirely inadequate to help and support or make contact with.

At this point in the process, I came into contact with the utter terror in me, a child within the war between the parents, with an aggressive, attacking father, and a mother whose way of handling it was to get hysterical or go to sleep, and who could not and did not protect me.

The experience of this terror took over my body ... I was shaking, verging on hysterical with terror. I had never consciously experienced this level of terror in myself before, in my body. I didn't know that this terror was there in me, the terror of the child in a war zone, in the war zone of the parents.

I remember once, when I was about ten years old, I was so distressed by the war between my parents that I ran out of the house in my pyjamas, down the street to the telephone box, and then I didn't know what to do. I didn't know who to call. It was late at night, I was distraught and near hysterical, and it was in a very small village in the English countryside. The only thing I could do was go home.

On reflection, after my process, I realised that this would have been exactly how I felt as a child when my parents were at war, and sometimes my father 'at war' with me ... totally inadequate to the situation and filled with terror.

The reactions we have to the external are to do with what is in us already.

Thank you, Mark Twain!

"It ain't what you don't know that gets you into trouble.

It's what you know for sure that just ain't so."

Mark Twain

A main challenge of trauma work is to sort out illusions from reality, and part of that is to see that much of what we are told about ourselves by our parents is just not true, or at best is only partially true. Without the means to access the earliest part of our lives, our time in the womb, and the time up until our Neo-cortex and cognitive memory have kicked in (about 3 years old), and even then, for many more years, we have to rely on what our parents tell us about ourselves.

"You were a wonderful baby ... you never cried!" Well maybe, but babies only cry in order to get their needs met, and if these needs are not met it is likely that at some point the infant gives up and resigns himself to this lack, and stops crying.

"You were a very difficult child ... you cried all the time, and you never slept!" Why would a baby do this? I find it so disturbing these days to see mothers with a child who cries, and the mother ignores the child. Babies cry for a reason. The cry of a baby means something ... it is often piercing in sound, and that is because the child's need is piercing for him.

So, our parents tell us these things, and since babies are hormonally primed to love the mother, and father, they also trust their parents. They have to ... there is no one else. Their existence depends on the child trusting those on whom he depends. The mother is the child's world. And so, we are primed to trust what our parents tell us; we don't even think about it ... we trust they tell us what is true, the truth.

But they don't, and it isn't. If we are traumatised then logically, we have to understand that our mother also is traumatised, and our father. Traumatised people tell the 'truth' that they can bear to tell, that doesn't re-stimulate their own trauma, the truth that they want to be the truth, their own fantasies about their own life, and consequently the fantasies they have about their child.

In all seriousness we cannot trust what our parents tell us about ourselves. It may be true, but it may not; it may be "what you know for sure" because that is what your parents have told you, and you trust them, but it may be a story that "just ain't so".

However, since we have this extraordinary method of setting an intention, of self-exploration, we can ask questions about ourselves, our experiences that we do not and cannot recall cognitively, either because these experiences were before our memory, or because we have had to split them off because they were traumatic. The residue of the truths of the early time of our life are stored in our body, in the cells and structures of our body, and we can access this truth of our own experiences through this enquiry method.

In fact, I would urge you to question everything about yourself, in order to find out the truth of who you really are. It's not that your parents were necessarily intentionally duplicitous. They may have been, from a cruel intent, but their answers to your questions will come from their own trauma survival instincts, to protect themselves, and perhaps with the misconstructed intent of protecting you. Question these stories always, and find out the truth about yourself.

Make no mistake, the one thing our parents for sure cannot tell us is what our own experience of something, of some event was. No one else can tell you anything about your own experience. If they try, be suspicious!

*

Here is another quote attributed to Mark Twain:

"It's easier to fool people than to convince people that

they have been fooled."

This is, in fact, the truth that parents are working on ... they can fool us with their stories and attributions about us, and because this happens when we are very, very young, and since children trust their parents, it is often hard for the enquiring person to give up on these stories and attributions. To give up on them means seeing the parents for the 'fooling' parents that they were, and that is hard. We have tied our life to these stories; we trust our parents because we love them, and to step into a world where we see how we have been fooled by them is not easy. It is painful and emotional as we bring into perspective this reality: they did not love me because they lied to me, they fooled me. But the pain is in having to relinquish the idea that, if I hold onto the lies, if I stay loyal to my mother's version of me and my life, perhaps my deep longing for her love will come to pass.

It is also a strategy that politicians and those in power use:

"A lie told once remains a lie, but a lie told a thousand times becomes the truth." Joseph Goebbels

Realising that you have been fooled changes everything. You are the only person who can know who you really are.

---------- ⟲ ----------

The big lie

Intention: "I want to accept reality"

The big lie: All mothers are innocent.

And so then, inevitably, it must be the child who is guilty.

*

In the case of the Trauma of Identity, the reality is that the mother did not want or love her child; that is her 'crime', and she is guilty of that.

This is a tough reality ... and it is easier for the child to decide it is his fault, and that he is the guilty one. If it is the child's fault, then perhaps he can do something about it, but this avoids the reality: he was helpless to do anything about it.

And it is easier for society to see it this way; the mother is innocent. Then society gets to avoid responsibility.

And it is easier for mothers and therapists to see it this way.

And Sigmund Freud came to see it this way, and developed psychoanalysis on this premise.

The child's urge to connect

Intention: "I want relationship"

The process went immediately back to the womb, so we know that the inability to gain a relationship is a symptom of the Trauma of Identity, the impossibility of a good relationship with the mother.

'Relationship' - "I am having to work very hard to connect ... it is a BIG EFFORT ... it is above my capacity."

The desire for relationship is more often than not the search for someone else to save us from our trauma and the disastrous lack of love and relationship with the one person we needed to have a good relationship with, our mother. This is not a good basis for relationship.

Solution: We need to develop a relationship with ourself ... which means we have to feel the pain of not being wanted and loved by our mother ... there is no other way.

Then, when you have developed a good loving relationship with yourself, you are able to have a good relationship with someone else.

The crash of narcissism ...

The diagnosis of the Narcissistic Personality Disorder is the only formal diagnosis that I think offers some usefulness to the IoPT practitioner, so before I start my essay, I will give this diagnostic information.

Narcissism is defined as:

> Narcissistic personality disorder (NPD) is a mental disorder characterized by a life-long pattern of exaggerated feelings of self-importance, an excessive need for admiration, and a diminished ability to empathize with others' feelings.[31]

The DSM V[32] categorises NPD as complying with at least five of the following criteria:

- A grandiose sense of self-importance
- Preoccupation with fantasies of unlimited success, power, brilliance, beauty, or ideal love
- Believing that they are 'special' and unique and can only be understood by, or should associate with, other special or high-status people (or institutions)
- Requiring excessive admiration
- A sense of entitlement (unreasonable expectations of especially favorable treatment or automatic compliance with their expectations)
- Being interpersonally exploitative (taking advantage of others to achieve their own ends)
- Lacking empathy (unwilling to recognize or identify with the feelings and needs of others)
- Often being envious of others or believing that others are envious of them
- Showing arrogant, haughty behaviors or attitudes

I would call the above description a grandiose style of narcissism, and in IoPT terms we are talking about the psychopathological end of the perpetrator attitude spectrum.

---

[31] Wikipedia
[32] Diagnostic & Statistical Manual version V

I would add another dimension that I will call 'humble narcissism'. The latter covers a kind of secret narcissism, every bit as consuming and grandiose in terms of extreme behaviour and personal perceptions, but in the form of a sycophantic and ingratiating attitude, exaggerated humility, constant apologising for their existence, excessively grateful and always asking permission, a display of worthlessness and helplessness that is not real, but enacted. It would parallel what we recognise in IoPT as an extreme form of victim attitude. "Everyone is against me, and I deserve it. I am nothing and no one can help me. I am, in fact, the worst person possible. I must please everyone to justify my existence. Nothing will ever be able to heal me from my trials."

Either way, both styles are impenetrable, and real contact is virtually impossible. To a great extent one is always interacting with an act, often an act that is quite seductive, engaging and charismatic, and that is why so often it is not properly detected or understood.

The consuming mother

In my book, Trauma and Identity (2021) I proposed something I called the 'Unwantedness Continuum', and at one extreme of this continuum I talked about a mother who is psychologically confused, and who wants her child for her own confused reasons that are nothing to do with the child. She projects her own fantasies onto the child. I also discussed what I called the 'consuming mother'. This concept means that the mother (in her narcissism) consumes the energy and liveliness and life force of the child, even to the extent of using the child's identity for herself, because she feels, underneath everything, that she is nothing and she has nothing of her own. Narcissistic mothers consume their own child to fill the underlying void and vacuum left to them by their own consuming mother. Therefore, narcissism is the legacy of a narcissistic consuming mother.

The narcissistic victim

The child of the narcissistic mother is left with nothing; all is taken and consumed and used by the mother to fill her own void of self, and the child grows up with an underlying conviction that they are nothing without the mother, and that their function in life is to save the mother from her trauma. This is the intent and end result of the enslavement of the child by the narcissistic mother, and it makes any form of separation or independent existence completely terrifying. Everything is drained from the child to the mother to fill her own emptiness. The child is forced into enslavement; a slave to the grandiosity of the mother, and slaves own nothing. As one client I worked with said "My mother ate me!", and as another said: "I have to get down on my knees and scrape the floor before I can meet my 'I'" where, in the process, the 'I' held the 'consuming' mother.

Because the reality of narcissism is that, underneath the attitudes and behaviours described above, there is nothing - no sense of self, of separateness, of an own life, own life energy and individual resourcefulness. Then the mother is seen as the only source of any kind of life, the only kind possible.

There are two survival possibilities for the child: the building up of a survival construct that follows the behaviours listed above, either the grandiose form ("I am wonderful like my mother"), or the 'victim' form ("I am nothing, my mother is everything"), and more often than not a combination of both, where one or the other may be the more commonly seen.

The task of the child is akin to the impossible tasks set by the wicked in children's fairy stories: the hero or heroine is set a task that is quite impossible, and then the impulse to achieve the task (heal oneself) is portrayed as someone like a 'fairy godmother' finally coming to their aid, or the hero/heroine finds some resource unknown before in order to complete the task. Healing is magic, and requires magical supernatural rescue, which of course in the real world, is impossible.

Healing the 'narcissistic wound':

"My mother is my life; I have no other"

The healing journey is challenging, and the separation from the mother takes time and is exceptionally painful and frightening. The notion that I cannot exist without her is real in the psyche of the child of a consuming mother, and the mother's continued use of the child as a prop to her grandiosity serves to offer some sense of existence to the person as an adult. As one client, who on occasion considered suicide, put it to me: "I wouldn't do it because I am frightened of causing my mother to be ashamed of me."

The 'crash' that I refer to in the title of this essay is the moment when the internal void of sense of self and existence is fully revealed, and the whole construct that has had to be adhered to crashes like a house of cards.

In that moment the whole charade of the mother and the relationship with her is glimpsed. The crash is the dark underside of the brilliant shining light of the narcissistic illusion, the reality of the vacuum within. This is such a terrible moment that, even though it is important and cannot be undone, it rarely resolves the problem completely. The loyalty to the enslaving mother takes time to resolve; to stand alone is terrifying and can only be achieved step by step.

The danger of being the whistleblower

The intention to heal is a threat to the system, the family, to the parents, even to society. Becoming a healthy authentic and autonomous being is a subversive political act, for which, in some countries and situations, people are forced to give up their freedom, and sometimes even their life.

Never underestimate the fact that, as much as politicians and governments say that they want everyone to live a good and healthy life, what in general they mean is that you should be controlled and only given 'freedoms' that fit with their own long-term goals. Because, whatever anyone may say, those who hunger after power over others have an agenda that is more often than not against the autonomy and self-authority of others, and is fuelled by their own trauma and their survival strategy of perpetration.

As much as a family that has harboured trauma and perpetrator-victim dynamics for generations, cannot tolerate someone in the family reaching out for something else - personal knowledge and healing - because it threatens the system, this also applies to societal systems.

To go into a therapy that understands trauma as we do in IoPT, is a threat as much to the status quo of society as it is to the family system. The whistleblower, whether blowing the whistle on the perpetration within the family or within government or society, puts him or herself in considerable danger. We have seen this with Edward Snowdon, who still has to reside in Russia because in the USA he will be tried as a traitor, and most likely jailed for the rest of his life, if not sentenced to death. And we can feel this in ourselves as we approach the issue of naming and revealing the truths of our family in the therapeutic setting.

To step away from the established, primarily perpetrator-victim dynamics, and the insisted upon 'reality' of the traumatised and traumatising family by speaking out loud truthfully about what has happened to us, and feeling our own pain, is more often than not seen within the family system as a terrible betrayal. And then the weapons family members may use against this 'whistleblower' are hatred, ostracisation, shame, blame and guilt-tripping ... all a form of 'killing off' the person.

Even if we do not actually tell our family the truth, (and I would certainly recommend that people think carefully about rushing to tell their mother and father and siblings what they have found and understood about the perpetration in the family), they will know anyway because of how different we are. The truth spoken, even within oneself, shows in how we then live our life. The traumatised family, the perpetrator family, cannot tolerate what they experience as such a betrayal.

Thus, we can see that becoming truly ourselves holds a considerable challenge ... we have to be willing to lose our family if necessary. And this means truly giving up on the deeply held illusion in all of us that if I hold still and quiet within the system, I will, eventually gain my mother's love.

Breaking away from the held 'reality' of perpetrator systems is always seen as a betrayal, primarily of the mother, and those family members (siblings etc.) who still hold to the family reality. All will blame this 'whistleblower', because it is too frightening for them to break free as well, and they too all hold the deep delusional yearning for the mother's love.

Taking oneself and one's trauma seriously may indeed, in very traumatised families, have potentially serious consequences, but this is the price of freedom.

The defence against the loneliness of existence

No one will ever see you, and value you, and love you, and understand you and your experiences, as you long to be valued, and loved, and understood. No one else can ever bridge that gap for you and fill this longing; no lover, no partner, no child of your own, no friend or teacher or mentor, no politician or government or social service or legal system, no therapist or IoPT facilitator can do this for you.

The title of Franz Ruppert's book: *All I want is to Live, Love and be Loved* … is the primary state of the newly created infant, of course, and if this doesn't happen at this earliest time of our life, these 'wants' then dominate our life; that is our trauma. What are we to do with that? How, then, do we live our life?

Of course, we must deal with and heal the traumas of not having this loving exchange as a child, these traumas of identity and love, but at some point, we will come to see the reality that the potential quality of that initial loving exchange actually from that moment on is impossible. No one out there can ever replace what we did not have from our mother. That is a bare truth, the reality, and if we look to these other places and people for this love, we will be disappointed. Others cannot do this for us.

That is not to say that love between people is not real and of value; it just isn't and can never be *that* love, and the problem is if we look to those other people to provide this impossible love, in the end we will be disappointed; and if we look to our children to provide this love for us, then they suffer their inability to do this for us; they can never love us enough, and that becomes their burden.

In my view this is beyond trauma. Even trauma, and its healing, the growing and strengthening of our 'I', all the activities that we do, every task we undertake, every experience we have, we cannot truly convey to anyone else. We can only experience it ourselves. We may describe a particular beautiful and deep process to a friend, but the translation from experience to account fails by being only a partial satisfaction. If we are looking for this primal loving connection in our relationships with others, it seems to me, it just cannot be.

This is what we have to deal with in the end, this existential aloneness. But whether this aloneness means we have to suffer *loneliness* is something else. In the end, the only person who can ever love you, appreciate you, understand you and share in the depth and beauty, and sometimes awfulness of your experience, is you. Our expectations and hopes that others can do this for us can only cause us more pain.

Perhaps to say that when one is as happy and secure in one's own company as one wishes to be in one's life, there lies peace. Then our interactions with others can be enjoyed to the fullness of the reality of what actually is, what these interactions can be, and that, then, is enough. There is love between people, between parents and children, but it can only be true as the love it can be, if we do not look to this love to recompense or replace that which we did not have.

To truly love oneself and be at peace with oneself, to value one's own experiences to the fullness that we know them to be, and understand that the sharing *is* pleasurable, even though it has limits, that I think is the true satisfaction of life. Then we can bridge the gap between ourself and another in a true and valid sense, without the disappointment of the unfulfilled longing.[33]

The experimental sentence

The experiment in IoPT is that moment when the facilitator makes a suggestion, most commonly in the form of a short sentence, for the client to say to one of her representatives. This experiment cannot be used until the underlying issue is clear, which is more likely to be towards the end of the process.

There are, I think, some useful things to say about this strategy in our work.

---

[33] . Perhaps read "No thought to the winnings", p???

1. The sentence should be short and encompass *only one idea*. For example: "I long for my mother's love."
2. The sentence content should attempt to reach underneath everything that has happened, to the core of the issue, directly to the trauma involved.
3. The sentence should be topical, in that it comes as a natural flow of what has happened so far, and it fits with the current situation in the process.
4. The sentence is only successful when the person is clearly themselves, i.e., through the process that precedes the experiment, the person has dissolved the confusion within her with her mother or anyone else in the process, and ...
5. The representative to whom she says the sentence is also clearly part of her, and they have established some reasonably good contact with each other.
6. The primary person to whom the client would speak the experimental sentence is the 'I', if possible (if there is an 'I' in the process and if there is some reasonably healthy contact between them).
7. The sentence can be said to another representative, particularly if there is not an 'I', but again good contact is important. Sometimes another representative shows healthy 'I' qualities ... that then could be the best potential connection.
8. Remember, healthy 'I' qualities include clarity and a good ability to be in contact; also, the representative clearly is an adult, not a child. Health is in the present ... it is the trauma from the past that makes us (or the representative) feel like a child.

The ultimate aim of the experimental sentence is to take the person to their deepest feelings, to the emotional pain of their trauma. The sentence aims to go to the heart of the matter, to the core of the trauma, and to invite the person to say the one thing they struggle never to say, for example that, even as an adult, there is still a deep childlike longing for the mother's love. This applies to the proposed sentence in point 1. above.

This kind of sentence, on the topic of the failed love between the mother and the child, addresses the deepest feelings related to the Trauma of Love. There are many versions of this sentence: substitute words such as 'want' instead of 'longing' and so on. As you explore the experimental sentences you will come up with your own versions.

Another very useful sentence to suggest at the appropriate moment, is the simple statement "I exist", or "I am alive", or any other statement that addresses the absence of support for the child's existence, the Trauma of Identity. The 'unwanted child' is caught between his natural desire to live and flourish, and his infantile (and mostly unconscious) need to fulfil his mother's wish that he should not exist. To say such a simple statement as "I exist" takes the person to the core of his Trauma of Identity. Saying such a sentence touches into the person's underlying reality of not being wanted, and having had to live a life of 'non-existence', while at the same time making a statement of freedom from the mother's secret injunction that he should not exist.

Other sentences are always primed to invite the person to say the unsayable, to state a fact that has not really ever been properly stated before. To declare, for example "My mother did not protect me", states a truth that could never be said before (Trauma of Sexuality, non-protection). The tendency is to prefer to accuse the more obvious perpetrator, as in, for example, sexual abuse by the father or other family adult, whereas the notion that the connection with the mother was not one of attention and vigilance on her part for the safety of the child, is often missed or glossed over.

Other examples of such sentences (and these are suggestions only):

> My father was not safe for me.
> My mother did not want me.
> My mother did not love me.

All of these kinds of statements help the person become increasingly in touch with the truth and reality of their childhood.

The direct purpose of the form used:

The distinction between whether to invite the person to say, for example "My mother did not love me" or "I long for my mother's love" is interesting. The first statement addresses the reality, the fact of the lack of love from the mother; the second addresses the person's own deep eternal longing. If we remember the basic issues of the Trauma of Love, the lack of love coming from the mother to the child, *and* the rejection by the mother of the child's own love for her, we can understand that, in effect, there are two stages of healing here: the first is the statement of the reality, and the second addresses the person's own experience of this deep rejection, this reality.

I think it is useful to think clearly about what we are suggesting the person say, and why.

When the timing is right.

When making such a suggestion to a person, we do our best to time it right, and to offer the sentence that really reflects the situation being addressed at that moment. Timing is crucial here, and often we will not get this quite right.

When the timing *is* right the person is put in touch with their deepest trauma pain, and can be encouraged to feel these deep feelings freely. This is a profound moment of healing, where the most painful feelings can be allowed to surface, and be expressed with the fullness and passion that they hold.

If the facilitator's timing is right, he will see this happen before his eyes. You can encourage the person to put their hands on their belly to focus their attention on this part of their body, because this is where the deepest feelings come from. Encourage them to trust their body, because their body is where the emotional pain is held, and their body needs to release from holding these feelings down, often in a very physical way.

It is likely there will still be moments of resistance, the survival impulses in order to keep the feelings down; a lump in the throat, the clamping shut of the mouth, holding the breath in an attempt to shut down the body, closing of the eyes. You can gently encourage the person to breath, to open their throat, trust the physical impulses they feel in their body. But do not over encourage; we need always to respect the person in the moment as to what is possible. Encourage up to the point where you might see what actually *is* possible right now. It may not be everything ... but it will be something. Always there is the tension between the natural impulse to expression and healing, and the survival impulse to suppress and maintain the status quo for fear of being overwhelmed.

Getting the timing right is a skill that may take some years of practice, to be able to see and sense the right moment. Making the connection between what is happening before you in the process, and the trauma that this shows, helps determine the correct sentence to suggest.

This is the sequence of the facilitator's journey:

- Understanding what you see. This takes time as the process unfolds. Do not rush. Perhaps we could say that the facilitator should start to really understand what she sees after about half an hour to 45 minutes from the beginning of the process, maybe sooner.
- Determine which trauma is the predominant trauma, whether the Trauma of Identity, the Trauma of Love or the Trauma of Sexuality.
- Choose the right moment.
- Make your suggestion.

If the timing is off ...

Very little may happen. But do not be discouraged ... there is nothing wrong; there is just information, and the information for the facilitator here is that this suggestion at this moment was perhaps too early, or not quite right. All the same, the words have been said, and in that sense the words and the implication of the words are 'out there' ... perhaps to be taken up again at some later moment. Never underestimate the ability of such seemingly unsuccessful attempts to resurface for the person some time after the process, and so be helpful to them.

The successful experiment allows for the whole process to culminate and find its own ending. In a sense, perhaps, there is nothing more for the facilitator to do. The job is done, and while there may be further things said between the person and their representatives, the shift is likely to have changed the experience of everyone.

When suggestions work, everyone is changed, enquirer, representatives, facilitator and observers. That is the beauty of this creative, collaborative process.

The infinite learning experience

I was introduced to this phrase by one of my colleagues, Sebastian. I liked it, so I thought I would share it with you.

Life is a continual (infinite) learning experience.

---◇---

The IoPT-informed person

The shift to becoming an IoPT-informed person is gradual ... and goes through many phases. It is the movement from the point of never having thought much about trauma as part of one's life, or of knowing one is traumatised but never really finding anyone who could explain and help, right through to realising that even history is likely to be re-written if we establish a society that is IoPT-informed.

Here's a question: do you ever now find yourself reading a novel, watching a film, even watching the news and before you know what is what, you suddenly have a flash of "this character/person is traumatised", or "that person is functioning from their survival 'I'"?

Here's another: do you now ever find yourself considering a painting, sculpture, or other work of art with which you are quite familiar, and seeing the impact on the painting of the artist's trauma. Does this then re-create the meaning and experience of the painting for you?

The other evening, I was watching a programme on television about D H Lawrence, the English novelist of the late 19th and early 20th century. A piece was being read from one of his novels: a man, at the bedside of his dying mother. I suddenly realised I just couldn't hear this piece of writing as it was meant to be heard, as it had been written. Instead, I heard it as an IoPT-informed person ... and it changed the story.

This is the result of a shift in consciousness that renders what one has seen and heard before obsolete. The man and his mother have a relationship over many years that, while recounted in the novel, never addresses the issue of trauma ... did his mother want him as a baby? And if not, doesn't that then influence completely their lifelong relationship, to the point now of dealing with her death? The IoPT lens can alter and inform what otherwise is a novel of its time; no knowledge of trauma then.

Once you truly become an IoPT-informed person it is like Alice stepping through the mirror. Everything, but *everything*, is seen differently.

Imagine, for a moment, some bit of history that you know, that you were taught in school, whatever your country or historic past ... just think about the details of this story for a few minutes. My history story is (which for the English is fairly typical) Henry VIII and his 6 wives. I have read many books about this period of Tudor history. Can you think about your bit of history now without thinking about the trauma involved and the resulting survival strategies, and the consequences for whatever happened next? How much does your IoPT lens change and inform in a new way what you have always thought?

To view our world and our history as an IoPT-informed person changes everything, and aids our understanding of things happening right now, from climate change to covid to Brexit (in the UK), to the economic challenges, Russia on the borders of Ukraine and moving to closer ties with China. Whatever it is, if you use your IoPT thinking and lens, see how the meaning of your focus is changed and your understanding enhanced by your IoPT perspective. What of the many massacres of history, the wars, the perpetration. The impact of trauma immediately reconstructs our understanding of the past. Imagine a history book written with the help of an IoPT lens. Even our understanding of history is likely to change when we include an IoPT kind of perspective.

Let's say we are 40 to 50 years into the future. I think the IoPT-informed Community will have grown. The 'IoPT community' perhaps quadrupled over the Covid era, since we all started working online ... and that was just within 2 years. Perhaps there then comes a point of critical mass, where enough people are IoPT-informed to the extent that IoPT thinking gently takes over the mainstream. Can you see what a cataclysmic consciousness shift that would be? It would be a force, powered by this critical mass of predominantly healthy 'I' functioning people, that would be quite unstoppable. In fact, I would go so far as to say that, rather than the need for protests and demonstrations, with all the potential perpetrator-victim dynamics and outcomes in order to attempt change, change (and health) would simply emerge. The more people who understand and are aware of perpetrator-victim dynamics, who see these dynamics clearly within themselves and in the world, the more people will find creative ways of stepping aside and not getting caught. Perhaps then, we might even dare to consider, those who would primarily function as perpetrators find no willing victims. Instead, we all manage to step aside.

"You may say I'm a dreamer … but I'm not the only one".

The reality is, once you really see and understand trauma your perception and understanding of yourself and everyone around you changes. History changes, and the future will change.

> Imagine there's no countries
> It isn't hard to do
> Nothing to kill or die for
> And no religion, too
> Imagine all the people
> Livin' life in peace
> You may say I'm a dreamer
> But I'm not the only one
> I hope someday you'll join us
> And the world will be as one
> (John Lennon)

Lennon tried hard to understand his world, but he was of his time. No mention of trauma then.

Franz Ruppert is of his time.

We are of our time.

———————— ⌀ ————————

The language of the mother

"I would like ... "

... is the language of the mother, replacing the more direct version, "I want". 'I would like" is grammatically the conditional form. It is cautious and conservative ... and it is polite!

It also holds the provision that I *may* get what I want, but I may not. Even, I could say, it is preparatory for disappointment.

We are conditioned in our society not to want, not to be so bold as to want. My mother used to say to me "'I want' doesn't get!" What a travesty of the child's natural impulse to want! This is the socialisation of wanting ... the pacifying of the child to the degree that the parent can tolerate.

"I would like ... " aims to pacify and calm the perpetrator. It is generally seen as more polite to speak in this way, but it is also a slip into dishonesty, and of course it also leaves open the possibility of not getting what we actually do want!

The pain of non-existence

I have often been amazed at the reactions of people exploring their own issues to the suggestion that they simply say to one of their representatives "I exist!" ... how often just the saying of this will put people in touch with the deepest feelings of their emotional pain. How the saying of such a thing resonates to the deepest part of the person's reality: "I do not really know that I exist". And how often I hear the person, after a visible struggle, say how difficult it is for them to say it. And even that they cannot say it. Such a simple statement ... and yet to say it can change everything.

We assume existence, because we are alive, but the unwanted child has had to split herself in order to survive not being wanted, and the only possibility then is a life of non-existence; "that is what my mother wants, and so that is what I have to do ... not exist in any meaningful way".

Existence is in the body. The notion of existence is just an idea. Existence is the experience of myself throughout my body and psyche.

Our trauma, particularly the trauma of not being wanted and loved, is so painful in the beginning of our life that, as part of our survival of this terrible reality, we numb our body and cut off our experience of this pain. And so, we cut ourselves off from the experience of existence. We, then, remain living in the twilight world of non-existence. The fullness of existence involves passion and liveliness; we can experience our toes and our heart, our knees and our belly; our needs and our wants are in the physical experience of existence.

There is no option in the end ...

If we want to be truly ourselves, we have to feel the pain ... there is no other way to freedom.

We can set as many intentions as we like, discover as much about ourselves as we can, but if we do not at some point drop down into those deep feelings that we have had to split off and bury in our body, we cannot in the end heal ourselves and free ourselves.

The price of freedom is to feel our pain.

The rationalisation of 'evil'

There seems to me, in ideologies such as capitalism and socialism, or any other 'ism', and perhaps I could say also in philosophy, an assumption of human rationality. However, I do not think we can talk about humans as being predominantly rational if we include the understanding of trauma that we have in IoPT. It is not possible, given the irrational nature of the trauma survival impulse, to assume that human motives and actions are necessarily always helpfully rational.

For example, for capitalism to assume that everyone is autonomous and quite capable of making their own individual success and achievement is manifestly not the case, hence the wildly out of balance situation we currently have in the world as to wealth and the ability to live a good and coherent life.

I am not knowledgeable about these topics, socialism, capitalism or philosophy, but what little I do understand does seem to assume a degree of rationality in humans in terms of our basic needs: to live, feed ourselves, have our children and stay alive as long as possible. But how does this explain such self and life denying phenomena as anorexia and bulimia, addictions, self-harming, cutting, suicidal tendencies, suicide and other activities of extreme self-suffering and self-harm, that go against the basic impulse to live and stay alive for as long as possible? For the most part such things are deemed 'illnesses', perhaps with a formal diagnosis, but without a particularly rational cause, and it is left at that.

The sufferer of a Trauma of Identity (and inevitably a Trauma of Love) struggles constantly between the impulse to live and live healthily, as against the impulse to fulfil the mother's desire that the person should not exist. Those 'illnesses' mentioned above are only rendered rational, it seems to me, through an understanding of the topic of trauma and trauma survival, which is absent in historical and present-day discussions of such issues and many other topics.

Our struggle over millennia to understand and rationalise humanity's tendency to violence and sadistic cruelty, not just in the incidence of wars, but also in our seemingly global tendency of cruelty and abuse to each other and to children, forced us to a concept of 'evil' as the primary explanation, and religious and psychological and philosophical ideologies and constructions as the explanatory solutions. But there seems no adequate explanation for this so-called 'evil', as far as I can see, other than the result of traumatisation: perpetration as a primary survival strategy of trauma, perpetration towards oneself and towards others.

Not only does an understanding of trauma explain what seems irrational about humanity, it also explains the tendency in some to function as 'evil', and, by way of amelioration, it explains our development of religious and other forms of ideologies in order to cope.

And incidentally, anyone who wants to talk about 'the patriarchy' as the cause of all humanity's woes must remember that all 'patriarchs' are the sons of traumatised mothers, with the resulting ability as adults to perpetrate against each other, women and their own children.

———————⌇———————

The representatives' limits

In the IoPT enquiry process we use other people to represent parts of ourselves so that we can see and understand the splits within us from our trauma. By doing so, and coming into contact with these split-off parts of ourselves, we can integrate some of our splits and become more truly who we are.

But as practitioners it is helpful to understand the limits of the resonance process: no one can heal anyone else's trauma, and as much as the representatives may show the enquiring person what is in him or her, and perhaps express strong feelings, in the end the representatives cannot do it for her.

The function of the representatives in the exploration process is to share with the person whatever their experiences are. The assumption is that these experiences are in fact the person's own split off and unacknowledged experiences drawn up from the person's unconscious by the phenomenon of resonance. In this way the designated person can access and share, through their experiences and feelings, what the enquiring person has split off and is unable to access.

Put simply, the representatives' job is to reflect to the person something of themselves that they may or may not recognise, but hopefully the information will help the person understand and know themselves better.

At times this includes a representative going into and expressing some deep emotions on behalf of the enquiring person.

But, just as children we could not feel and express feelings fully on behalf of our traumatised mother, to save her and protect her from her trauma, so too the representatives cannot in the end feel and express the true trauma feelings of the enquiring person. The very best the representatives can do is show the person what is in her, what feelings are waiting to be experienced and expressed by her when she is ready. This is the limit of the representatives' ability: the representative cannot do it for the person, they can only show the person what is in him or her.

If during a process the expression by a representative is particularly deep and seems fulfilling, in my view this is because the representative draws on her own trauma situation and, perhaps we could say, takes the opportunity to feel some of her own split off trauma feelings. There is nothing wrong with this, but the practitioner knows that for trauma to heal we all have to express and experience our own feelings; we cannot use the representatives to do this for us.

The representatives of parents

I think you can trust the representative of a parent, but you cannot trust the parent. There is a difference.

In the IoPT process the representative of a mother will share her experience with the enquiring person in different ways, each one, to an extent, reflecting what the enquiring person can actually bear in the moment.

- The representative may speak as the actual parent might ... not sharing anything that the enquiring person does not already know. In fact, in the resonance enquiry process this is rare, but it does on occasion happen, perhaps more often when the person chosen to represent the parent is new to the resonance phenomenon, and unsure how much she can trust what comes up in her.

- What is more common in the resonance process is that the representative may speak as the parent, but because it is a resonance process there emerges more truth as to who she really was. For example, the resonance can own the underlying hatred/fear/absence/disinterest etc. Thus the resonator speaks as the mother, but with the awareness of underlying issues that may have been in the actual mother, but would never have been spoken by her. Usually, these issues are recognisable by the enquiring person, but perhaps are out in the open for the first time; never said, allowed or given the status of truth and reality before.

- The third category is again slightly less common. This is where the person resonating can say things about the mother as the resonator of the mother, *but not as the mother*. In this instance the resonator will speak as herself *about* her experience as the mother. In such a situation it seems that there is an allowance in the process for information to be forthcoming, but it cannot be owned by the 'mother' in the process. The actual mother would not speak, but the resonator is able to speak on her behalf from her experience as a resonator.

These distinctions are subtle, but I think interesting and useful to think about.

And we need always to remember that the mother we are faced with in the process is the mother as she is held in the person's psyche; she is that mother that the child could not defend him or herself from as an infant, not so much the here-and-now mother. The trauma is the issue, and the trauma happened long ago.

———— ࿇ ————

"There was nothing to want ... "

Intention: "I want intimacy"

'want': "I, as the baby, didn't make the decision [not to want]; *there was nothing to want.*"

'intimacy' (to the Enquirer): "I don't feel much ... I look at you. You are very beautiful ... I want to copy you, my hair like yours. I can't say: do I want to be you or do I want to be like you? I am very young."

A perfect description of identification; the survival strategy of the Trauma of Identity. In this process the mother was in the enquirer ... or in 'intimacy' ... it was hard to tell; the enmeshment was so tight.

The substitute or hidden 'I'

If there is not an 'I' in the intention, or even if there is but no one represents it, there is, even so, always an 'I' somewhere in the process. 'I'-ness is always there, but because of the circumstances at the earliest time, the child's 'I' may have had to be hidden away as a primary survival strategy: it simply was too dangerous even to have a submissive 'I' ... having no discernible 'I' was safer.

It is often the case, particularly when working with people new to IoPT, that there may be no 'I' in the sentence, and even if there is, it is not thought of by the person as having the importance that we, in IoPT, know it has.

Grammatically the word 'I' is the subject word, and stands for our experience of subjectivity, being a subject of our life; whereas objectivity, being treated by others as an object rather than as the subject of our life, equates to trauma. 'Me' and 'myself' are the object words grammatically.

The absence of an 'I' in the sentence, and even if there is an 'I' in the sentence but the person doesn't not choose to have this 'I' represented, in the first place demonstrates a lack of understanding of

IoPT thinking about the 'I' and subjectivity. It is often the case that, after seeing others set intentions, and coming to understanding something of IoPT thinking, the person will put an 'I' in their sentence, and perhaps give this 'I' a representation in the process.

Even so, there can still be a question as to whether the person is simply following 'the form' of IoPT, and the underlying issue that downgraded 'I'-ness to non-existence may still be there and active. However, if represented, the 'I' resonance will give information on this.

The absence of an 'I' can indicate the impossibility of having an 'I' and any form of subjectivity, as a child in his family. To say "I want" is an expression of healthy subjectivity, and this may well not have been allowed or possible as a child. The 'unwanted child' would struggle to hold onto his or her 'I-ness'; safer, perhaps, to silence, suppress, or even obliterate, any sense of 'I-ness'. The mother's 'I' and her wants prevail.

But I think there is always an 'I' in the process. Look to the representatives for the qualities of 'I'-ness, qualities of a healthy 'I': clarity, intelligence, calmness and adultness. The healthy 'I' is always adult; it is only the traumatised or survival 'I' that comes across as a child.

The threshold

There is a threshold that comes, not in every process we do, but perhaps two or three times in one's overall journey of setting intentions.

This threshold is the moment we stand on the edge; something has happened, something said, some gap in the world. We are looking into the void; we can't control our breath, our stomach heaves and a convulsion starts, low down in the belly, the same movement as if we are going to vomit, but it isn't vomit. It is the body, beginning to release.

The convulsion continues upwards from the deepest part of us and, if for this brief moment of our life we let it happen, we do not distract, we trust ourselves, the convulsion waves up our body into our chest, our mouth and throat open, and the energy rises up and up and up, and eventually if we go with this pure physical purge, it is like a wave crashing on the shore, and perhaps we release a sound from the depth of our being, an animal cry, the wail of the trauma released at last. The convulsions of emotion take on their own volition, and our body releases the deepest tears, convulsive tears ... perhaps our body shakes and thrashes in the emotion, in the release, what has been held for years is allowed its expression, and nothing, ever, is the same again.

Most of our intention process do not end like this, but they all contribute to this moment when it comes.

———————oᴧɔ———————

The Traumabiography

The Traumabiography consists of four sequential and consequential trauma experiences:

- The Trauma of Identity - not being wanted
- The Trauma of Love - not being loved
- The Trauma of Sexuality - not being safe
- The Trauma of Becoming a Perpetrator - causing harm to others

For each trauma, the subsequent trauma is both a consequence and a solution.

The first thing to understand is that traumatised children have traumatised mothers. A mother who was not herself traumatised would be unlikely to cause trauma to her child. However, since in my view we are all traumatised, such a situation is extremely unlikely. In order to understand this better you might first want to read the essay entitled "A necessary digression" (p.13).

The Trauma of Identity is about existence ... and not being wanted by the mother at the beginning of our existence. The survival strategy for this trauma is identification.

The Trauma of Identity means that I cannot exist as me ... I cannot hold onto my identity, as new as it is in terms of my experience. I cannot hold on to the reality of myself as separate and distinct from my mother.

Instead, in order to have some vital contact with my mother, I have to split off my own experiences and traumas and live according to my mother's ideas and attributions about me; her will and wishes prevail. I have to identify with the external and split off my own internal sense of myself. That is identification, the survival strategy of the Trauma of Identity.

The mother, in not wanting and not seeing her child for who he actually is, then, defines the child's identity, but this is not who he is. This is the survival constructed identity that complies as necessary with the mother's version of who the child is.

The Trauma of Love is the inability to establish a loving connection between mother and child at the beginning of life. If the baby is not wanted, it follows that the mother does not love the child, so the Trauma of Love is an inevitable consequence of the Trauma of Identity, and in my view happens pretty much at the same time. To not be wanted is to not be loved.

There are two parts to this Trauma of Love:

1. The mother does not want the child, so she does not feel love for the child.
2. The mother also, then, rejects the child's natural instinct to love her. She rejects the child's love which is all he has.

So, a natural loving exchange cannot exist, and the child suffers.

The Trauma of Love, for the child, is also a 'solution' to the Trauma of Identity. The child can do nothing about the terrible situation of not being wanted at the beginning of her life. It is a devastation that the child is far too vulnerable and helpless to manage, and so causes a trauma and psychological splitting to survive.

But the Trauma of Love offers some hope for the child. If I cannot gain love from my mother, perhaps there is something I can do ... love her more, take care of her, protect her, understand her, become a better child, become more what I perceive she wants from me, distort myself to try and fulfil her desires. There is hope.

There is no hope with the Trauma of Identity and it is so unbearable that the Trauma of Love seems to offer some hope for the child that she can do something to gain the mother's love. This longing for the love of the mother, and the endless attempts to establish that, then become the substrate of one's whole life if not addressed.

The Trauma of Sexuality

There are two parts to the danger of a Trauma of Sexuality for the child:

1. The absence of vigilance on the part of the mother - the child's safety is at stake.
2. The presence of sexual confusion in the mother, and also the father, that can lead directly to the enactment of sexual exploitation of the child.

The Trauma of Sexuality is a consequence of the Trauma of Love (and therefore of the Trauma of Identity) in the following way: If the mother does not want her child, and so consequently does not love the child, she is not going to be a safe refuge for the child. Her ability to sense any distress in the child is numbed, and her ability to protect the child is therefore compromised or absent.

A mother who wants her child, whoever the child may become, and loves her child for who he or she really is, would be attuned to her child, and would have the ability to sense distress or changes in the child that would result from some danger or unpleasant experience. In addition, such a child would have no impediment to turning to the mother for refuge, help and safety should something untoward happen. The child would trust the mother to believe her and protect her. So, the danger for the child is there in the absence of vigilance in the mother.[34]

There are two forms of the Trauma of Sexuality

1. Sexual confusion of the parents, due to their own trauma, that clouds and influences the familial context.
2. Sexual trauma that is enacted.

The ultimate danger for the child of sexually traumatised and confused parents is that the child becomes an object to the parents, for living out their own sexual traumatisation. The most severe form of this is the

---

[34] It is, in the psychotherapeutic world, extraordinary how often, in the final telling of the truth of sexual abuse in the therapy, the fact that the child could not tell the mother, or father (in the case of the perpetrator as someone else) is not seen as an important symptom of the relationship between mother and child. In general, the fact that the child could not tell the mother of the abuse is seen as to do with the child, her shame and distress, rather than as to do with the mother. The Traumabiography tells us something different: it is the mother who fails the child; it is the mother who is the ultimate perpetrator.

sexual use and exploitation of the child, and both parents are involved in this. Sometimes both parents perpetrate sexual practices on the child, and in other situations the father does and the mother colludes, either by ignoring what is happening or by, in some way, offering the child to the father or other potential abuser, and sometimes it is the mother who is the actual sexual perpetrator to the child. Either way, the parents should be the attentive guardians for the child, and if any kind of sexual exploitation occurs both parents are involved. It cannot be otherwise.

Trauma of Sexuality as a solution to the Trauma of Love:

A very common way in which sexual abuse may happen within the family is through the child trying to find a solution to the Trauma of Love, in a family that is shadowed by trauma and sexual confusion. If the child cannot gain good, loving contact and attention from the mother, she or he is extremely vulnerable to sensual and/or sexual exploitation by the father (or in fact anyone else who shows some attention to the child). The young child turns to where there is a possibility of attention, but if the father has his own Trauma of Identity and Trauma of Love, on some deep level he also is looking for the absent love of his mother, and the danger is his own need for love and attention gets projected onto the child, and his own sexual confusion becomes acted out with the child. The child becomes a confused object for the father in his search for his absent mother love; the child becomes a potential 'mother' for the father, and sometimes a substitute for his estranged relationship with his wife, the child's mother. Such is the confusion of the Trauma of Sexuality.

In my view, historically this confusion has been compounded by the origins of psychoanalysis and psychotherapy, where the child was seen as the perpetrator of the 'innocent' parents by having aggressive sexualised fantasies of the parent as described in the Oedipus Complex.[35] All the child wants is connection and love, to feel that he matters to someone.

There is a further complexity here in that, if the mother herself is traumatised and sexually confused, her choice of partner or husband,

---

[35] The Oedipus complex, in psychoanalytic theory, is thought of as a desire for sexual involvement with the parent of the opposite sex and a concomitant sense of rivalry with the parent of the same sex; a crucial stage in the normal developmental process. Sigmund Freud introduced the concept in his Interpretation of Dreams (1899). (Sourced from Encyclopedia Brittanica).

the father of the child, will also likely be similarly confused. It is extremely unlikely that a woman who, herself, has come from a sexually confusing and even sexually exploitative background, would come together with a partner as father to her child who is not similarly confused. Or, to put it the other way around, a man who has a relatively clear psyche, and an absence of sexual confusion himself, is unlikely to end up with a woman who is severely sexually confused. So, a situation where, in the absence of care by the sexually traumatised mother, the father is safe for the child, is probably unusual.

The Trauma of Becoming a Perpetrator

In fact, from the beginning, we are forced to become a perpetrator to ourselves. We are, through the experience of the Trauma of Identity, forced to split off our truth, our true identity, and comply with our parents' wishes, attributions and ideas about us. As a result, we are forced to behave towards ourself as our mother behaved towards us. The 'internal critic', for example, was initiated by her. Self-hatred was instigated and installed in us by our mother's hatred of us; if we were not wanted, self-hatred and self-abuse were the solution. We align ourselves with our perpetrator mother in our self-perpetration. We behave towards ourself as we were taught to in our initial survival of not being wanted.

There is no reason at all that any creature would hate itself; there simply is no point to self-hatred in the realm of life's impulse simply to continuously recreate itself. It is only humans that indulge in self-hatred and self-harm, and it is the inevitable result of traumatisation.[36]

So, perpetration against ourselves is already familiar in us from the start. Even the natural response to traumatisation, splitting off our experiences and feelings, is a perpetration. It is not what we want, but it is what is forced on us.

---

[36] I am not entirely sure about this, but everything I read on the internet tells me that self-harm amongst other creatures is seen only in the context of human influence, for example in a zoo. Whether there is actually self-harm within the realm of other species untouched by humans I am unsure. However, I do not see the logic of self-harm in the natural environment. To harm oneself seems to me to be pointless in nature. The primary necessity is to protect oneself from attack from others and to defend one's territory, and then self-harm is illogical.

Perpetration is a primary survival strategy of traumatisation and in certain circumstances we will enact harm on others in order to protect ourselves from our own trauma feelings. Self-perpetration then becomes perpetration towards others. Whether it is perpetration by enactment of harm, or perpetration by neglect, or perpetration by classifying others as perpetrators and feeling victimised by them, causing harm to another is a primary form of trauma survival. Hurting someone else deflects us from our own feelings of vulnerability and helplessness. Perpetration helps us not to feel our own pain, but instead forces someone else to feel pain.[37]

When we hurt someone else, the natural result within us is to have feelings of shame and guilt. If we allow these feelings, they provide us with a healthy impulse to do something to right the wrong, to address our perpetration and act accordingly. However, if we suppress these feelings, we harm ourselves; we split ourselves further from ourselves. This is the trauma of becoming a perpetrator to another.

Each time we hurt another, we are faced with the uncomfortable feelings in ourselves, which, if repeatedly suppressed, result in an escalation of splitting and self-numbing. We end up with less and less healthy feelings, and less contact with ourselves, and an increasing ability to harm others. Perpetrator dynamics are constantly escalating.

The experience of perpetration is both powerful and empowering. It is a diversion from feeling our real helplessness and vulnerability, and instead allows us to feel powerful and strong, and we can easily become addicted to this drug of power. The more we have to suppress ourselves, the less alive we feel, and perpetration then becomes the answer. Power is an addiction. The end result is the 'psychopath' or 'sociopath', addicted to power in order to have some sense of life in a self that is massively suppressed.

Anyone who desires power over someone else is a perpetrator, and is burying their healthy human feelings of guilt and shame.

ᐟᐟ

---

[37] Victim attitude as a survival strategy: We have in IoPT theory the survival categories of 'perpetrator' and 'victim attitude', but the 'victim attitude' is another form of perpetration. To live as a victim does indeed distract us from the underlying reality of our original victimisation, but it is still a perpetration against oneself and others.

Thirty years of therapy

A woman came to an online group session and said that she had done thirty years of therapy, and she thought that IoPT might offer something else. This is something the IoPT practitioner hears from time to time.

Thirty years of therapy is a long time, and one wonders at that. Isn't therapy supposed to resolve people's problems? Isn't the idea that therapy helps? And yet we know that analysis for many people becomes a lifelong regular venture, a seemingly never-ending needed support for life; something the person becomes increasingly and endlessly reliant on. "My therapist says …" is a common thing people say. Think of Woody Allen's films where part of the comedy is the endless psychoanalysis as a constant backdrop.

This woman set an intention, and in her process her representatives could not look at her, and could not connect with each other. One, a man, started to relate in harsh and excruciating detail experiences of sexual exploitation, all of which the woman confirmed as having been her experience. This went on for a while; the 'I' representative switched off her video and would not come back.

I realised that I began to feel protective of the representatives, particularly the man who by now was lying on his desk and continuing to describe in detail various horrible sexual experiences.

I do believe that the IoPT practitioner has some responsibility for the wellbeing of those who offer themselves as representatives, not in an overly caretaking way, but this feeling of protectiveness for them in this moment was by way of an alarm signal to me. On the one hand I wondered what on earth had been going on in her thirty years of therapy that this should all be coming up in such vile detail now, and on the other I thought I had to stop it. So I did; I paused the process.

Then I asked the woman what she wanted from her process. This was a question she had difficulty answering, but one of the representatives, the male representative did; he said he wanted joy and love and laughter.

This woman knew everything; every detail that was spoken by the representative, she already knew. So, what is the point? The most important thing in the IoPT exploration process is to find something new, some new perspective, new information, new feelings - a shift of some sort. There must come something through the enquiry process that the person did not have before. That is the point. If that doesn't happen then the work fails.

This woman wanted to be heard and to be believed. She had spent her years of therapy wanting someone else (the therapist) to validate her existence. She used her sexual exploitation as her identity, as loudly as if she wore a badge; "I am the victim of extraordinary sexual exploitation ... that is who I am".

Usually in our work, the enquiry process is useful in order to discover that which has been split off, forgotten or denied, and in this way people who have split off their terrible sexual exploitative experiences, can come to know what was done to them and complete the sense of who they really are. This is the point of a process that is called, intentionally, an 'enquiry process' or a 'self-encounter process': to find out personal experiences and information that have been split off, feel the feelings, the pain involved, and from there complete their sense of themselves and free themselves from the burden of their splits and their often self-persecutory, survival strategies. Our identity is the accumulation of everything that has happened to us, including that which has been split off, forgotten and denied, whether 'good' or 'bad'; nothing missed out. That is who we are, and that knowing of who we are comes from within, and does not require validation from the outside, from a therapist. The aim of the IoPT enquiry process is to complete the puzzle of who we really are, to fill in the gaps, find the truth amidst the mis-directions and lies that abound, address those experiences that were so awful we had to split them off and deny that aspect of ourselves, and feel the split off feelings.

But this woman already knew it all.

So, when I asked her what she wanted from setting this intention, eventually after struggling with the idea of wanting something at all, she said that she wanted to be believed, and she asked me if I believed her. This was my response:

"It is not important whether I believe you or not. The question is: do you believe yourself?"

The need for a therapist or other external authority to affirm your experience is the externalisation of your identity; the other (the therapist), then, is required to confirm your very existence. This is the root of identification, the primary survival strategy of the Trauma of

Identity and, I would say, the major flaw in conventional psychotherapy. The conventional therapist may become the mediator of the client's existence; they unknowingly collaborate with the survival strategy of the Trauma of Identity - and are in danger of becoming the source of identification.

At the end of the process the woman said: "Every therapist I have been to has said I have to go to the trauma [the sexual trauma] and describe it. That's what I have always done. I have always been looking for someone else to believe me."

For thirty years this woman had been re-traumatising herself in the hands of psychotherapy, reliving these awful experiences without respite. The only identity she knew was her sexual trauma, and for thirty years she had had this affirmed back to her by the external. The awful reality of the underlying traumas of not being wanted and not being loved and protected by her mother had been successfully avoided in favour of a constant re-living of the sexual trauma. The perpetrator mother gets to escape and the client stays in her trauma, a constant in the here-and-now victim.

To practitioners ...

Your greatest teachers are your clients.

You will learn more from your work with others than in any other way, except your own personal IoPT explorations.

In every process that you facilitate, be determined to learn something you did not know or see before. Be alert to this great source of learning. This is how Franz Ruppert developed his IoPT theory, and it is how you can become a good IoPT facilitator.

Trans-generational trauma?

Intention: "I want to be"

At the beginning of the process the 'I' representative said: "There is some trans-generational trauma here".

If this is said by one of the representatives, we, as facilitators, cannot afford to ignore this. If we do ignore it, we may be in danger of missing an important entanglement across generations. But the question then becomes, what does the 'I' mean, and who perhaps from the past is necessary to bring in as a representative?

In IoPT we prefer not to go too far from the enquiring person herself in terms of looking into the past, and we are right to do that. Bringing in people from past generations too often becomes a distraction from the actual issue, and even bringing in a representative for the mother, while at times useful, can often become a distraction away from the person herself and her original representatives. No one can heal anyone else's trauma, and only you can heal yours. How much you need to know from the past in order to do that is questionable.

But if the person's mother has a Trauma of Identity and a Trauma of Love with her mother, and her mother also has a Trauma of Love from *her* mother ... neither mother nor grandmother were able fully to hold onto their own identity and being, and each then looks to their child with entangled eyes, and this creates great confusion in the present person.

In most processes it is quite easy to see where the mother element is, in the original representations, or in the person herself. Representatives often say that one or other of them seems like the mother, and sometimes a representative will say that the enquiring person herself seems like the mother.

In some processes, as the facilitator watches and tries to see the presence of the mother somewhere, she may see 'motherness' everywhere, in all the representatives, and also in the client herself. If we listen carefully to what the representatives say we may find 'essence of mother' in *how* things are said, and *what* is said. Here are some examples from this actual process:

- The representative for the word 'be' says to the enquirer: "You don't want me!" Of course, we could hear this, perhaps correctly, simply as it is ... "You (the enquirer) do not want me (one of the enquirer's parts)." This is perfectly valid, and may be borne out by what happens next. But we could also hear it as a child speaking to her mother: "You (the enquirer seen as mother) do not want me (representative as child)." In this case the confused representative for the word 'be' would be a child seeing the enquirer as her mother, and we could see this 'motherness' in the client herself.

- The representative for the word 'I' says "I don't trust 'be'." Mistrust between representatives is a strong sign of such a confusion. Who is who? ... and which representative holds the 'mother influence' in this lack of trust?

- The 'I' says: "I want so much more ... I'm not satisfied!" These are not the words of a small child ... these are words of 'motherness'. It is subtle, of course, but somehow these do not seem the words of a child. The traumatised child would not speak in this way ... the child just wants contact, but already knows this is not possible, and has learned quickly not to ask, and certainly would be unlikely to say "I'm not satisfied!" That is a statement of rebellion few very young children can voice until they are much older.

In such a confused situation where the mother seems to be everywhere it is useful to bring in a representative for the mother, to see if the representatives then are able to be clearer as to their sense of themselves and their relationship with each other, and with the enquiring person herself.

If this doesn't work, and the mother representative herself seems also very confused, perhaps fairly young and not sure who she is, then it might be a time to bring in her mother, the grandmother.

The reason we bring in such representatives from the person's past is because they are already in the person's psyche, as evidenced by the overall confusion, and it may be that bringing in these extra representatives clarifies things and allows the original representatives to just be themselves and be more in contact with the enquiring person.

The notion of 'trans-generational trauma' is of course real. My mother's trauma (her traumatic relationship with her mother) is what I, as a child, inherit in terms of how my mother is with me, and we can get clearer about this by seeing in the process how the mother and grandmother are, and the information that comes from the representatives. But to go further than this, in my view, is unlikely in the end to be helpful. The *only* reason to bring in representatives of people from the person's past is for information, and there is always a question as to how much of this information is really necessary. Perhaps see the next essay entitled 'Understanding as a Substitute for Love'.

Understanding as a substitute for love ...

Intention: "I want to be free"

If I cannot give my mother love because she has always rejected it, I can, instead, try to understand her ... to understand why she doesn't love me, and why she rejects my love. I can offer her my understanding as a substitute for my love, which she rejects; but in the end this becomes a constant distraction, and is not a route to freedom.

I can persist in looking into her past, trying to know what her trauma is, trying to understand her lack of interest in me, believing that there is something in her, perhaps in her past, and that if I can just discover it then I will understand her, and she will love me.

Maybe I set intentions that, rather than explore me and my issues, in fact rather wish to explore her, learn more about her. Her existence, history, trauma and reality, then, is more important than mine. Or it may even be the case that I cannot distinguish between my experience and hers, my existence and hers. Perhaps my intention is subtly and unconsciously the intention that she would have chosen ... I can do it for her! I can free her from the trials of her past, her childhood! She will respond to my loving understanding of her traumas!

In addition, how can I really have a sense of my own existence if she, in herself, doesn't feel her existence, if her trauma causes her to lack a sense of life and freedom? Can I exist as a child if she doesn't have any experience of existence herself? What right have I to exist if she cannot feel and glory in her own existence? Would my real experience of existence then cause her shame and, worse than that, leave her to struggle on her own with her experience of non-existence?

This is the nature of the child's love for his or her mother. "I will do anything for her and then, in the end, I will gain her love."

In this way I can avoid the disastrous reality that she doesn't want or love me, but I remain entangled with her, and I am not free.

Freedom comes from facing the truth, and that means turning away from trying to understand and love your mother, and turning instead towards yourself, understanding and loving yourself. That is freedom.

Valuing our tears

Intention: "Why do I submit to authority?"

The explorer cried when she understood that the 'authority' she feels forced to submit to is her mother ... and then she distracted herself from her own honest and valid feelings, to wipe every tear away and blow her nose, clean herself up.

Even in the wiping away of our tears, the wetness of our feelings, we are obeying our mother. Our tears are part of our expression of ourselves. Why do we have to wipe them away so vigorously? Why are we so ashamed of our feelings and the visible expression of them?

My mother used to say to me "Stop crying! Blow your nose!" She couldn't bear to see me crying; it made her feel helpless ... and even ashamed. I was evidence of her incompetent mothering; I, in my pain, in that moment, showed her up in her helplessness. I, then, began to feel ashamed of my tears.

My first husband was a photographer, and when he was in his twenties he stayed with a family in New Zealand, and, with the permission of all the family members, he photographed them, as they were, whatever was going on. Not so many smiling faces in this body of photographic work. This was a family that was prepared to show themselves to a stranger, just as they were. Distress and tears at the kitchen table were allowed to be seen and captured in dramatic black and white. Images of hurt and pain, despair and hopelessness, a mouth open and eyes clamped shut in unhappiness; tears and snot streaming out or trickling down a face. Nothing exaggerated, nothing forced. The family got so used to him being around with his camera that they showed him the beauty of their very real feelings. Of course, there were many moments of happiness and joy in this family, but his main interest was in what most of us keep private. He stayed with them for about six months and produced the most extraordinary body of work. No pain was unfit to be seen, and no tears were brushed aside in shame or embarrassment.

I tried to find a good photograph online to demonstrate this, but all the photos I found looked staged to me, not real. Unfortunately, I am not in touch with this man any more, otherwise I would show you one of his beautiful photographs.

Why are we so ashamed of our sad and unhappy feelings? We put on a face of happiness in most of our photographs; we shut away our pain with shame. I wish I had the confidence and skill to do such a project myself.

The explorer, through her tears, said: "I have to love the part of me that still loves my mother ... that is also a part of me."

We don't need IoPT clones!

Do not use IoPT as an identification, as a survival strategy!

Everything you have experienced in your life is part of who you are as an IoPT practitioner. Become a real IoPT practitioner. Become yourself as a unique IoPT practitioner.

Yes, copy if you must in the beginning. That is many people's learning form ... it certainly is mine ... like children, learning by mimicking our parents ... identifying with our parents' ways and thinking.

But if IoPT theory means anything at all, we can become true individual-thinking, autonomous IoPT practitioners.

We live in the present ...

And trauma is always in the present, no matter how many years ago it actually occurred. The traumatised split off parts are frozen in time, frozen in the moment of splitting, frozen with the emotions unexpressed, un-felt, unknown. That is why so often one or more of the representatives in a process, experiences themselves as a child, even in the womb. That is the moment the trauma happened and that moment is frozen in time, cut short and left. There is still a pained and traumatised baby-in-the-womb split off in the psyche of many of us.

I have noticed when I suggest to someone I am working with that he say something like "I long for my mother's love", that sometimes people change the present-oriented sentence to the past ... "I longed for my mother's love", as if speaking about themselves long ago. But this is one step of avoidance of the real pain that we live with every day of our life.

The representation that is shown in the Intention Method process through the representatives and their experiences, is the current here-and-now state of our psyche. Everything shown happens now, every moment of our life. To put it in the past already distances us from the heartbreak of what is shown.

To say "I wanted my mother's love" distances us from the present reality that is stated in the sentence: "I want my mother's love." It is this present statement that pulls us into the actual reality that we live every moment of our life.

What can we do for peace?

" …everyone you meet is fighting a hard battle."

Socrates

A healthy psyche, a healthy 'I', does not hurt another person, because to hurt another automatically hurts the person as well.

The healthy 'I' knows this. The trauma survival 'I' forgets it.

Definition of a perpetrator: someone who harms or causes hurt to another, directly or indirectly, consciously or unconsciously, flagrantly or secretly.

Perpetration is the primary survival strategy of traumatisation. I hurt another so that I do not feel my own vulnerability and helplessness, my own trauma.

If I hurt someone else, however, I have to deal with my own shame and my own guilt, and that hurts me. If I bury my shame and my guilt, this hurts me further, and prepares me to continue to hurt others as well. This is the inevitable cycle of increased perpetration.

If I hurt someone else, they are victimised and, as part of their trauma survival, they may turn perpetrator and hurt others. Thus, in my action of hurting someone, I am complicit in any hurt that person may cause another. So, if we hurt another without recompense or acknowledgement, we may be sending another perpetrator into the world.

Each harmed person has to make a choice: do I focus on my hurt, my own trauma, or do I avoid my hurt and my trauma by hurting someone else?

What President Putin does at this time[38] is hurt many people, and by this action he escalates hatred in the Ukrainian people, and the desire to hurt back. So escalates the perpetration cycle.

To hate is to hurt. The child does not come into the world with hatred, but only with love, the desire to love and be loved. That is the nature of life as it is within the child and all creatures. The child and mother, under

---

[38] Ukraine war, 2022.

healthy circumstances, are hormonally primed to love each other. Life requires this love in order to flourish.

Hate comes in from the outside. The child learns to hate from a hating parent; that is the only way that hatred comes. Hatred from the outside becomes the contract, the connection, instead of love, and this can only result in self-hatred. The unwanted and hated child can only survive by agreeing to the mother's terms: "I hate you, so in order to gain connection with me you must hate yourself."

The hated and self-hating child judges and criticises themselves, continually hurting themselves, psychologically, emotionally and often physically. The hated and self-hating child grows into an adult who, in order to deal with and avoid their own internal self-hating process externalises this torture and hurts others. The experience of power from hurting another perhaps makes the person feel better, less helpless and vulnerable, for a while, but power is an addictive drug. Lack of power connects us with our trauma, and then we look for someone to whom we can express our power again so that we can continue to avoid our vulnerability and helplessness.

Hatred is against life. Do other creatures hate? We might think that a creature hates in order to gain territory or safety. Then hatred might have a use, but I think this is actually healthy aggression, not hatred. I am pretty sure no creature hates itself, no animal, plant, or tree, or insect hates itself. It just does not serve nature.

No other creature bothers itself with hate. Even the predator does not hate his prey; and prey does not hate the predator. They know and understand each other and the necessities of life. They may use aggression in order to gain their food and other needs, or to protect themselves, but hatred is different. Hatred simmers and grows with each experience of perpetration against us, and with each act of perpetration we make against another. Hate never achieves a useful result; it only propagates more hatred.

To live in peace, we have to recognise our self-hatred and our ability to hate others, and to do this we have to feel and know our vulnerability and our helplessness, and we have to know that in others. It does not help to hate someone like Putin for example; when hate enters us, and fuels our actions, we fail, because we join the perpetrator-victim dynamics.

So, what can we do?

The only thing we can sensibly do is acknowledge and take seriously our own deep trauma. If we do not do this then our perception of the world is distorted, and the invitation to join the fray and the hatred grows.

If we externalise the solution onto governments and those in power we are lost again into the world of hatred. But if we work to clear our own psyche of the distortions and survival tactics we have had to develop since birth, then we strengthen our healthy 'I', and it is only from a healthy 'I' that we can have the clarity to make a move, take action that will not result in further destruction.

We need to make the internal move from this:

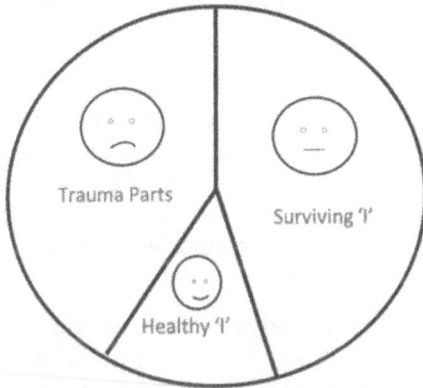

... where our healthy 'I' struggles and the survival 'I' dominates, and our traumas remain, secluded, split off, alone and forgotten ...

... to this:

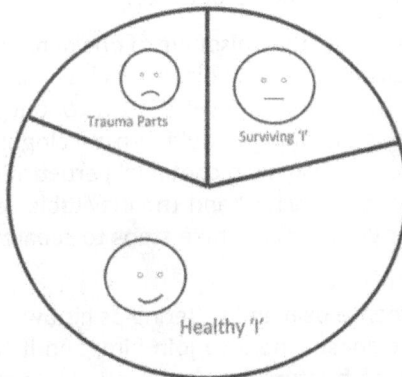

... where our healthy 'I' is strengthened, we have fewer unresolved traumas and our need of survival strategies is inevitably less. The healthy 'I' knows what our trauma is, and knows our trauma survival strategies. The healthy 'I' recognises when our unresolved traumas are triggered and, instead of collapsing into our survival strategies of hatred and harming, can find more useful solutions, set further self-enquiry intentions, and resolve to take ourselves and our trauma seriously.

Then we can stay calm in the face of adversity, see reality as it is without the distortions of our survival 'I', solve problems with clarity, intention and purpose, recognise those problems we cannot resolve, and find ways to move forward anyway. It is only from our healthy 'I' that we can make good decisions that do not complicate the situation further.

We are only ourselves. We cannot solve the world's problems, and we cannot do anything useful if we do not see reality clearly, if we fall into survival emotions of hate and passion, blame and accusation. The healthy 'I' above all is realistic. Yes, we live in a world where perpetration is rife, but we cannot change this by force or further perpetration. We can only change ourselves, and thus, perhaps, we can influence others by our being.

Socrates said: "Be kind, for everyone you meet is fighting a hard battle." Even Putin fights with his own internal demons, his own helplessness and vulnerability. He projects all of his own self-hatred onto the Ukrainians at this time, but we are all complicit. We have all happily ignored the reality of his trauma. We have over the years given him the benefit of the doubt, and refused to see the reality of the potential of his trauma perpetration. We have ignored reality that stared us in the face. We did not recognise the perpetrator.

In the UK Putin authorised the poisoning of one of his adversaries in the beautiful city of Salisbury, with a poison developed in Russia, that also killed an innocent bystander, and yet the UK continued to trade with Russia, always hoping that things would turn out alright in the end. Over the years Putin has got away with continual perpetration, and it is only now, with the Ukraine invasion (and the inevitable real threat to the rest of us) that our governments take steps to separate from him and his Russia.

Yes, he causes immense pain and suffering as his own survival strategy of perpetration. It doesn't help to join him, and it hasn't helped to ignore the threat of his further perpetration. He would not stop, because he feels a victim, and perpetration is his strategy of avoidance. Each act of perpetration that he makes, and then sees that other governments still work with him, still ignore his potential to perpetrate further, strengthens his idea that perpetration works.

Yes, if I were a Ukrainian living in Ukraine this would be the hardest situation I would ever be facing ... yes, I might kill or harm for my survival, but in the end that is the way of the perpetrator if I do not feel the ultimate pain of my actions, my own shame and guilt, my own tragedy. I cannot say what I would do in such a situation as the Ukrainians find themselves in right now. Thankfully I am not, and since I am not, the most useful thing I can do is try to see the situation clearly, think for myself from my healthy 'I' what is best for me to do, realistically and within the realms of my ability.

Everyone I come across is dealing with this dilemma, and perhaps the least I can do is remember that everyone I meet is fighting a hard battle.

What is love?

" ... what seems to make sense is that the first encounter between egg and sperm is an act of love, and not of struggle."

(Ruppert, 2021)

Love is the lifeforce. Literally, love is what urges life to be, the force of life in all things. The impulse of all creatures and plants is to exist, to grow, to become, to flourish, if possible, is the force of life, and this 'force' is love.

Love is an experience in your body and psyche ... it is the result of the release of hormones such as Oxytocin and Dopamine.

We dramatise love as something special, something sought after, to aspire to, but it is there, right at the beginning of our existence, if allowed. It is there even now, in the most loveless and love-lost situation; even so, love is there, in the very existence of you.

The tragedy of the human species is what we have done with love, what we have had to do with love. Our creative intellect has displaced love for what it really is, and we have then had to make up ideas about love, most of which are illusions. We have had to do this because real love experience is difficult for the traumatised. In order to understand why we have lost our love we have to go back to the beginning of us, and understand why we, of all species, are so uniquely vulnerable to trauma.

Why are we humans so prolifically traumatised?

In our evolution, at some point, we began to rely on our intellect in combination with our physical powers. We began to think, and imagine other realities, other possibilities. We became creative. We learned to imagine, and to lie. Creativity is about lying, in the broadest sense of the word; we could think about and speak about something that wasn't in that moment true, but from this creative act, could become true. We began to plan and design things that didn't exist until we thought them and planned them and designed them and created them.

This is what distinguishes us from other species; we began to explore our thinking, to use our brain, and create unimagined realities. We started to use our psyche in increasingly specialised ways. We started to rely on our intellect and our creativity.

> "Every cell is a living organism consisting of matter, energy and the possibility of processing information. In this way, all living cells have a psyche and can learn from their experiences."
> (Ruppert, 2021)

All species, whether plant, insect, mammal, reptile, have a psyche that is developed to the level needed to satisfy their basic needs: gaining food, safety, specific environmental conditions (warmth, cool, dry, wet etc) and the reproduction of their life form. Even a single cell has a psyche. Even species with no detectable brain have a psyche. Mycelium is thought of as 'the brainless decider'. It makes millions of decisions every day, but has no brain. You do not need a brain in order to have a psyche.

However, humans, over the millennia, have increasingly relied on their intellect to solve problems and create the things needed, specifically the neocortex part of our brain, the most recent and most sophisticated part. This urge to imagine, create and explore has contributed to many consciousness shifts. Enforced evolution and adaptation to environmental changes also cause shifts in consciousness and increased intellectual ability. This is the same for all species; one thing we see at the moment with climate change is that some species are already adapting to the changes, while some cannot and so, will inevitably die out.

Our focus and reliance on our intellect, at the expense of our attention to our emotions and love and somatic experiences, was expressed most clearly by Descartes' aphorism "I think, therefore I am". We have favoured and relied increasingly on our intellect, to the extent that we have come to disregard our emotions and the truth that they offer. We can lie and create myths and stories about life with our intellect, but our emotional and somatic existence does not lie. We have come, over time, to mistrust our emotions, and the sensations in our body, and rely instead on our intellect, but this has also meant a confusion and loss of reality in many situations. The intellectual creative reality has, at times, taken on more validity in our thinking than our physical, emotional and resonance ability. This is one reason why we find the representation resonance process we use in our IoPT practice to be a bit mysterious and seemingly unexplainable. We tend to regard it as weird, but it isn't. All creatures use this sense, resonance, every moment of their lives, in order to fulfil their needs to find food and to keep safe from predators.

The cost to humans of our intellect is our excruciating vulnerability for many years as a child ... and this is where trauma comes in, and the loss of the life force of love.[39]

Trauma and love

For all other creatures the life force (love) is a simple issue. It is just there, and supports all creatures to grow and develop in their own unique way according to the genetic information of their species. The mother sheep[40], as soon as her lamb is born, will clean him and encourage him to find the nipple and start sucking. The lamb, once born, struggles to stand almost immediately, and then searches, follows the smell, to find the mother's nipple. As the lamb grows there is a

---

[39] You might want to refer to the essay entitled A necessary digression (pp13) to understand this better.
[40] I keep sheep where I live, and from my house I can watch them as they birth and care for their young.

constant maintenance of contact between mother and offspring; as the lamb explores and moves into the wider world around him, he will call to his mother, and she will answer. These impulses are life-preserving and prompted by the hormones of love.

But the traumas we humans experience because of our unique vulnerability at the beginning of our life, more than anything else, restrict the free-flow of love. In the beginning, the in-utero infant is hormonally primed to love the host, his mother, and hopefully to receive hormonally primed love from her. This is nature's way of giving the baby a good start in life, and is expressed in the title of Ruppert's latest book: *"I want to live, love and be loved"*. This is the simplicity of our existence. This free flow of love between mother and child, in its intended form, offers the most positive start to life.

However, a mother who has suffered a trauma of connection with *her* mother as a baby will be likely to traumatise her child. She is separated from the free flow of love, and cannot offer this for her child. To feel that life force of love fully would force her to confront her unresolved trauma feelings. We can only experience this life force of love when we are fully in our healthy 'I', and only if we can *stay* fully in our healthy 'I'. The moment that the underlying trauma is re-triggered we split and go into our survival strategies in order to distract ourselves from the terrible emotional pain of our trauma. The experience of love cannot remain once we are in our survival strategies. The experience of love puts us in touch with our body and our deepest emotions, but the survival 'I' cannot allow this, because these deepest emotions always include the unresolved trauma experience. So, to feel love properly inevitably puts us in touch with our unresolved trauma.

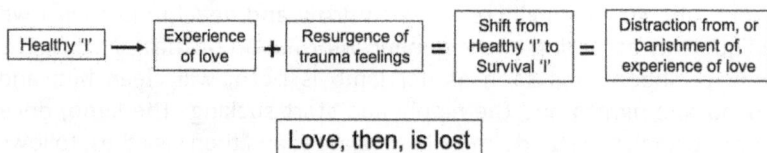

| Healthy 'I' | → | Experience of love | + | Resurgence of trauma feelings | = | Shift from Healthy 'I' to Survival 'I' | = | Distraction from, or banishment of, experience of love |

| Love, then, is lost |

The survival 'I' does not know, nor allow, love. It is simply too dangerous to feel this emotion for the trauma survival 'I', and it must be distracted from, banished, obliterated and forced into a delusional aspiration that can never really happen, the chase after the 'love ideal'.

If the mother is compromised in her ability to connect with her child lovingly, she is also compromised in her ability to receive the free-flowing life force of love from her child. She cannot open herself to receiving this love from her child and so rejects him in his being, or distorts this gift from the child into something that does have meaning for her. For example, she may distort the child into the source of love she should have received from her mother, and the child becomes the surrogate mother to his own mother, sometimes even before he has exited his mother's body and physically separated from her. In the mother's intellectual ability to create delusional realties to protect her from her own trauma devastation, she will distort her relationship with her child in a myriad of ways, and the infant has no defence against this. He has to accept the current reality as it is and survive as best he can. Already his life force is compromised or even lost. Love is lost, and another traumatised parent comes into being as the child grows up.

I think that this kind of trauma has been with us humans for millennia. This could explain the phenomenon that all IoPT practitioners find in their practice: everyone is traumatised. To be sure, some people are much more traumatised than others. The level of traumatisation is variable. For example, if the current generation of people who become IoPT-interested and informed, recognise that they are traumatised and take it seriously and set intentions to heal themselves, their potential to traumatise their own children will be less. Hence, theoretically we could heal all of us in three or four generations (see essay entitled Healing the world! page 43).

And what of love?

What have we done with this love, our life force?

To know when it all began generationally, is perhaps impossible, and certainly is not necessary for us to be able to live a good life. We cannot heal ourselves by looking into the past, except insofar as we can understand the traumatising ability of our parents. We can only heal ourselves by exploring ourselves. The solution is within us, not out there.

The only thing that stops us from living a good life is the delusions about love that we create.

When one is living from one's healthy 'I', there is love for oneself. When one is living from one's survival 'I' there is not. If there is love for oneself, then one is truly in touch with one's original life force, and from there comes love for others.

<hr />

What is the solution?

It is useful for us to spend a little time thinking about what we are doing when we start a personal enquiry, and when we come to facilitate someone else in their self-encounter process; the purpose of the IoPT process in relation to the theory of IoPT.

I have four answers to this:

1. Integration of the splits

The overall purpose of IoPT work is to integrate what has been split off because of trauma.

If we understand that surviving trauma required us to split off the trauma experience, then in our psyche we are split. This means that the solution would be to integrate the split off parts, feelings and emotions. So, we can say that the overall purpose of the enquiry process is to integrate that which has been split off in our psyche. This is shown in the enquiry process when the representatives, the parts of the person, all come into good contact with each other and with the enquiring person. This is not always possible, and so we come to point 2.

2. To understand something new, a shift in perception

Each intention set, and the resulting process, is an enquiry into ourselves, and so we can say that the primary purpose of the enquiry session is a shift in perception and understanding, a shift in one's relationship with reality. There must come something new, something that has not been known, seen or understood before, otherwise there is no point to the session. Each shift in perspective, moment of insight, new understanding is a step in the direction of integrating the splits.

3. An opportunity to face the truth and feel the feelings

Always, in the end, we have to feel the feelings, and facing the truth is the primary trigger to allowing these feelings.

4. To become more truly who we are and live a good life

The answer to all our quests is within us, not out there, and the IoPT enquiry process offers us the means to explore ourselves, find ourselves and achieve these results, thereby finding a way to live a good life, and live in peace with ourselves and those around us.

What kind of future do we want?

This essay attempts to imagine ways of establishing and maintaining high standards of professional practice and adherence to ethical behaviour for practitioners of healing disciplines in the 21st century. We are, I think, in new territory with this topic. Certainly, since Covid, many practitioners of different disciplines have started working online, which has opened up their working world to a global practice. I imagine this raises many questions for professional associations that they have not had to think about before.

In the past this 'holding of standards' has most commonly been done by the establishment of a 'professional association'. The association then, sets standards, instigates 'accreditation' procedures and develops post-graduate strategies to hold good standards over time, along with attempts to establish a 'code of ethics' to ensure good ethical behaviour between individual practitioners, between practitioners and their clients, and in relation to the general public.

There are fundamental reasons why this form of 'holding' is the antithesis of the basic principles of IoPT. Accreditation, for example, requires practitioners to submit to the opinion of others – supposedly more experienced and able to make such assessments – before they are officially allowed to practice. This method contravenes the basic IoPT principle of autonomy and self-responsibility. In fact, it follows the basic survival strategy of the Trauma of Identity, by forcing the practitioner to an identification with others' views, just as the unwanted child had to identify with the mother's wants and biases as to who the child actually is. This 'outsourcing' of the authority for one's identity onto others is an undermining of the person's own ability to make clear decisions from their healthy 'I' for themselves ... in effect it assumes the inability or fragile ability of anyone to do this for themselves.

However, in favour of the accreditation procedure is always the question of how aligned the person can be with their healthy 'I' ability in order to decide on their own fitness to practice. Accreditation, as contrary to basic IoPT principles as it is, does attempt to give the public some marker that they could possibly rely on when choosing a practitioner. However, there are further problems with this method. Accreditation provides a boundary, after which the practitioner is deemed to be 'safe to practice', but our personal and professional lives bring about all sorts of changes to us, and thence to our practice. This ongoing process of living must require a form of continual assessment, and most psychotherapy associations require, for example, an annual 'Continual Professional Development' (CPD) submission and a re-accreditation procedure every five years or so. For IoPT practitioners the question then becomes: How does a practitioner decide in any one moment that they are fit to practise, and how can the public be able to rely on practitioners' quality of practice? I will discuss this more below when I come to talk about IoPT peer groups.

Another issue comes with the establishing of 'codes of ethics', that in general take the assumed basic values and principles of the community of practitioners and attempts to put them into bullet-point 'rules' or 'guidelines'. Then all members of the association are required to adhere to these guidelines, and infringement has consequences, sometimes quite severe. However, even the making of these 'rules' and 'guidelines' is a major challenge because such rules in practice so often invite questions and variations that continually alter and manipulate the original rule. Even a simple rule on something that on the surface looks very clear, for example against having an intimate and/or sexual relationship with someone with whom one is working or has worked, raises many questions. The UKCP[41], for example, states as one of their guidelines for ethics and professional practice that the practitioner should 'Not have sexual contact or sexual relationship with clients'.

---

[41] United Kingdom Council for Psychotherapy.

However, this seemingly simply guideline invites many questions as to the following:

- What constitutes an intimate and/or sexual relationship?
- Should we ban all such relationships?
- Is it always exploitation, or could it sometimes be a genuine potentially loving relationship?
- Should we impose some kind of time-limit? For example, if one meets the person in a workshop, how long after the workshop could be deemed a reasonable lapse of time to pass before one could engage in intimacy?
- Or should we say that if you work with someone, even only once, then that person is off limits for life?
- If a practitioner happens to meet the person who they really feel they want as their life partner on a workshop they are facilitating, what then do they do? (In such a case in the UK more than once in the past a psychotherapist has had to relinquish their profession in order to be with their chosen life partner.)
- What is exploitation?
- Is it really exploitation?
- Is it always exploitation?
- And if we say it is exploitation, are we diminishing our clients' own ability to be self-responsible and make adult choices, such as who to have an intimate/sexual relationship with?

It is easy to see that both of these attempts (accreditation and holding to an established code of ethics) which attempt to control the quality of work and the behaviours of the community of practitioners, are what we in IoPT would probably prefer to avoid.

But at the same time, there are issues that we will have to face, the main ones of which are:

- How do we maintain the clarity of the theory that we have, how it is practised and how it is taught?
- How do we hold practitioners' behaviour and quality of work to the basic standards that IoPT theory infers?

Our theory, at first sight, looks simple to understand, and easily applicable to oneself and one's own experience, but those of us who have been working with IoPT and Ruppert's ideas for many years know so well that the theory is actually complex, and has a depth of life understanding that is not possible to see at first sight. To say, for example, that a person was not wanted by their mother (Trauma of Identity) is an intellectual concept until we penetrate the individual's experience of it. Each person's 'unwantedness' is unique and individual, and the emotional response to becoming aware of it is entirely the person's own response. To practise this work is complex and demanding, and no less is it to teach the work.

We may say that the principles and basic values of IoPT will support our practice, and yes, that is possible to an extent, but there are problems with this. One example is that the person new to IoPT, who sees the benefit and logic of the basic theory may, rather than wrestle with the underlying complexity look to other disciplines to support them, but this may deflect them from grappling with the complexity.

We may also say that the underlying values of IoPT will hold us as practitioners in terms of our ethics, our behaviours towards our clients and members of the general public, and towards each other, but we must also remember that, because we are traumatised, there is a perpetrator impulse in all of us. This impulse may show itself at moments when we feel challenged, when we are triggered and flee into our survival constructs. There are issues as to how we talk about each other in private, and how we deal with a client who tells us something critical about another practitioner, how we manage moments when another practitioner does something we feel critical of; how we respond to others' ideas and style that do not conform with our own. We, all of us, are human, and we are all traumatised, and as such realistically we are all vulnerable to moments of unethical behaviour.

So, how can we work with these issues and find a way to do this without going down the controlling and hierarchical route of a professional association? It is hard, and perhaps in the end we may find it impossible. After all, already there are 'licenses' issued to some practitioners.[42] Already our community is split into the licensed and the non-licensed. What are the consequences of this?

---

[42] Professor Ruppert has already issued 'licences' to certain practitioners. The questions we have to ask ourselves here are these: if we agree to this 'licensing', who else can 'license' anyone, particularly after Ruppert retires or is no longer available to us, and what does it actually mean? Would there be any form of common consensus as to what the license implies, and if so what, and who decides this? And who decides on the issuing of licenses, and what does having a licence actually require of the licensee in terms of quality of practice and ethical behaviour?... and so on.

These are not easy questions, but I do believe we must face them, and probably face them now rather than wait until we are forced into something we do not want.

*

What can we do?

I would like to offer a solution to some of these dilemmas. My solution covers two things: one is the membership of peer groups and an understanding of the possible functions of such groups; and the second is a basic principle of ethical practice that can be developed and held to within each peer group.

1. I would suggest that every IoPT practitioner or student practitioner becomes a member of, or creates along with some others, a small working peer group, not more than six or seven members, and that these peer groups meet on an average of every four to six weeks, either online or in person. This is not a rule, but perhaps it could be strongly advised. In fact, it could be beneficial for practitioners to become members of more than one peer group … this enhances the cross-fertilisation of ideas as a member of one group takes something of what they have learned in that group to another group. Through this means we could have a global constellation of many peer groups that are all in some way in contact with each other.
2. That all peer groups are varied in the level of experience, i.e., that members recognise and welcome practitioners who are more or less experienced than they are, and do not end up all functioning at a similar level. Members then learn from each other in different ways; the less experienced may learn from the more-experienced, and the more-experienced person gains skill in talking about theory and practise, and may have some of their established assumptions questioned.
3. That we understand and follow the basic functions of being a member of a working peer group, as I will set out below.

Functions of peer groups

At present, from what I hear, most peer groups are oriented around a setting in which they can practise their skills, i.e., do intention processes with each other. However, I would propose the following additional functions of peer groups:

1. To intend to create an environment that runs on basic IoPT principles of respect, valuing and support of individuality and autonomy.
2. To use the Intention enquiry method to clarify any of the issues that may arise within the group, including many of the following.
3. That the members care about the group and each other and their development and commit to attendance over time.
4. To think about and establish the group's own ideas about confidentiality for their working group.
5. To gain personal support from each other, particularly if someone is struggling with painful understandings from their own personal work.
6. To share their successes and failures and problems in their work together in a helpful and emotionally supportive environment.
7. To study the available texts together to improve their understanding of the intricacies of the theory.[43]
8. To think about connection with others in the wider IoPT field, and perhaps to invite someone with greater experience to 'visit' the group for a meeting occasionally, or sometimes perhaps to combine with another peer group for a meeting.
9. To discuss issues of personal 'fitness to practice', which for each practitioner may change over time depending on personal life circumstances. The value of 'fitness to practice' then becomes one of personal and collaborative consideration, rather than something one decides on one's own, and the group together then take responsibility for holding standards of practice. It is useful to set intentions to clarify such issues.
10. To maintain a continuing awareness of issues of ethics and values as to interactions with each other, and with other members of the IoPT community, with clients and with the general public, thereby developing a personal and group sense of responsibility for holding a high standard of ethics for the whole IoPT community. Again, setting intentions can help to clarify such issues
11. To consider how to creatively manage and deal with any infringements of what one would think of as ethical behaviour between practitioners, and between practitioners and their clients, and with the general public. The group then provides a resource for thinking

---

[43] There is already a 'reading group' of practitioners who are focused on reading the texts available together, and to help with understanding.

collaboratively how to address such issues, rather than seeing them as others' problems and colluding with potential perpetrator-victim dynamics. If, for example, a group member, has a complaint, or is complained against, the group together will find creative ways to support the person to find a healthy solution that would hopefully allow for a peaceful settlement all round. Setting intentions is a good way to gain clarity for such issues. (See below for an example of dealing with a complaint about a practitioner.)

In this way we might be able to maintain an ethical community with high practice standards.

A working definition of ethical practice for consideration:

Some years ago, I had occasion to think about a general definition of ethical practice, and I came up with the following:

Ethical practice involves continual self-reflection and scrutiny combined with committed dialogue with colleagues.

Resolving ethical issues

I would suggest that the foundation to resolving ethical issues is the commitment of all practitioners to such continual self-reflection and scrutiny in collaboration with colleagues, and an open commitment to dialogue and setting intentions to gain clarity.

Here is an example of managing an ethical issue:

Some time ago I had an email from someone I didn't know, asking if there were an IoPT association in the UK to which she could make a complaint about a practitioner. And if there weren't, should she then make a complaint to the practitioner's psychotherapy association? It seemed that the practitioner was an 'accredited' psychotherapist and a member of a professional psychotherapy association. Could I help?

I spent a couple of days thinking about this and discussing it with several colleagues. I then wrote back thanking her for her email, and expressing dismay that she should have had such a difficult experience that was causing her to want to make a formal complaint.

I told her that there was no association for IoPT and some reasons why. I said she could of course approach the practitioner's psychotherapy association, but that it was doubtful whether it would have sufficient knowledge and understanding of IoPT work to be able to make a suitable response.

I then suggested she contact the practitioner and ask for a meeting to discuss face-to-face what she had not been happy about. I added that if she felt in need of support to do this she might see if she could find someone within the field to act as a mediator. I added that I would be happy to help in this capacity if necessary.

Finally, I said that I hoped she could get appropriate satisfaction and that she might, in spite of her difficulty, find good ways of benefitting from the work in the future.

A week later I had an email back thanking me and saying that she had arranged a meeting with the person concerned. I replied saying that if I could help further to get back to me. I heard nothing more.

*

I include this story as an example of how we might be able to work without a formal code of ethics and procedures for dealing with complaints and grievances by a commitment to dialogue. Of course, in this instance the person was able to take the suggestion in the manner it was intended, and this is not always going to be the case. It also stands on the assumption that any practitioner who values their work and practice would always be willing to engage in such a meeting with a complainant.

I think that there are two parts to resolving difficulties that arise:

One is a commitment as a practitioner to face-to-face dialogue (in person or online), when possible, perhaps mediated by a third, uninvolved person. This has been well demonstrated as helpful in The Truth and Reconciliation commission work in South Africa and Ireland.

And the second: when resolution in the way that one would wish seems unattainable, is agreement to the 'isness' of things as they are. This avoids the escalation of perpetrator-victim dynamics, where in the end there are no winners, only losers.

The aspiration of always, if possible, attempting to resolve issues by inclusive and committed dialogue, combined with self-reflection and consultation with colleagues in, for example, a peer group, seems to me a good way to go and, if resolution is not possible, a realistic acquiescence to things as they are as a way of avoiding perpetrator-victim dynamics.

In the conventional professional association, an infringement of one of the ethical codes is often followed by grievance and complaints procedures, and at times cases are even referred to the legal courts. This involves a long journey of escalating perpetrator-victim dynamics.

There is also here, I would suggest, a deeper potential for trust in the rightness of things; that, in the end, people are responsible for their own lives, and it is often the difficulties and stumbles that we make in our lives, that provide us with the greatest opportunities for learning. We all make mistakes, and learn along the way. Sometimes if someone politely points something out to us, we suddenly see it in another way, and can take another step towards greater wisdom and better practice.

"Who am I?"

This was the intention

You do not need your parents in order to know who you are.

In fact, they are the ones who forced you to forget who you are.

*

Who or what you are not

First to say: only you can ever know truly who you are. No one else can do this for you.

You are not:

1. Your mother ...
2. Or your father
3. Or anyone else in your family
4. Or your ancestors

5. Who anyone else tells you you are
6. You are not the stories your parents and others tell about you
7. You are not the stories you have had to make up about yourself as a child to fill the void or protect yourself, or explain yourself
8. You are not how you show yourself through your survival strategies. You have utilised these strategies in order to get to adulthood, and while these are your strategies and as such are a part of who you currently are, you are much more than that
9. You are not your symptoms, which are only your survival strategies calling your attention to your trauma, to heal yourself

The answer to the question "Who am I?" is within you, in the recesses of your unconscious, in the actual experiences you have had from the moment of your creation; your own trauma, your own survival, your own reality.

You are, and were, right at the beginning of your life, a separate and independent being, the result of one egg and one sperm coming together in the spark of the creation of life, *and* you were also dependent on the external context of your world, your parental situation.

The fall from this beautiful innocence is that at the beginning of your life you were also dependent on another to sustain your life ... and that is where your troubles began.

Who owns the womb?

This came up in a process where the 'mother' representative clung onto her womb and wanted to withhold the womb from her child. The actual mother had attempted to abort her child, and in the session the representative for the mother kept saying "the womb is mine!" So where does the child live for nine months? Who owns the womb during pregnancy?

Of course, in an ideal and untraumatised situation this question would not exist; the womb belongs to both in their common endeavour to support the creation of new life. But in the traumatised situation of a child who is not wanted, and even the mother attempts to abort the child, she is saying to the child: "This is my womb and you are not welcome here." Then the child has no home.

Who owns the child? There is another question.

In a healthy situation a parent may refer to 'my child', 'my daughter', 'my son', but while this indicates the nature of the relationship, it does not necessarily imply ownership. The parents are responsible for the child's wellbeing and safety until the child can do this for himself, but that is responsibility, not ownership[44]. The parents do not own the child; as the child approaches adulthood, the parents are relieved of their responsibility for the child.

In the animal world, in the wild, the mother assumes this responsibility naturally, as best she can, until her offspring can manage on their own; then her job is done. For many creatures, once this job is done, mother and offspring separate and sometimes never see each other again[45].

"Why am I still struggling?"

Intention: "Why am I still struggling?"

Because there is something, still, you do not want to see.

---

[44] Ownership: the act, state, or right of possessing something. (Oxford Dictionary)
[45] For example, the Snow Leopard, and other big cats.

Will and I – (1)

If you align yourself with the positive life force in you, your fundamental will to live, then you have the resources to gain your own 'I'.

You need will to gain your own 'I' …

And you need a 'healthy I' to use your will in a healthy way.

Do not assume in your process that your 'I' resonance is a healthy 'I'.

In fact, if there is an intention to be done, then the 'I' in the intention, if represented, will always be confused. It can never be a fully 'healthy I', because if it were, there would be no problem in the first place, and no intention.

'Will' and 'I' – (2)

Musings on the plane back from Singapore. Blog post 05 August 2019.

This story arises from an understanding of the impact of early trauma, what it means to have a confused 'I' without access to one's own 'will':

'Will' is helpless without the clear-sighted purpose of a healthy 'I'. She (or he) flails around, looking for guidance and purpose; she tries this and that without success or meaning.

She is energy without direction, fuel without a match, hope without a plan.

A confused and entangled 'I' squanders 'Will' on hopeless endeavours, on bullets and barbs, petty quarrels and castles in the air, momentary amusements and endless disappointments, useless protestations that achieve nothing.

The confused 'I' wants the unattainable, believes the impossible and expends precious energy pursuing nonsense rhymes. Like the Red Queen of Alice's Looking Glass World, the confused 'I' runs as fast as she can, only to remain on precisely the same spot, breathless and exhausted, piling confusion on confusion.

And 'Will' looks helplessly on, praying that one day 'I' will take a hold of herself, use 'Will' and ask the question: who exactly am I?

The confused 'I' doesn't see 'Will' as her own, as the child of herself, patiently waiting direction and purpose. In her confusion 'I' assumes 'Will' is the enemy, either lacking sufficient power to rescue 'I' from her confusion, or as a perpetrator always wanting something from 'I'. She may even grow to hate 'Will', not seeing her patience and fortitude, but confusing her as belonging to another, as the cause of 'I's confusion and pain. Like a helpless child 'I' waits for rescue as 'Will' watches from the grey shadows. And nothing changes.

'Will' can change nothing without 'I', and 'I' can do nothing useful without 'will'.

And perhaps one day 'I' spies 'Will' as she sits patiently to the side.

Perhaps, for once, 'I' looks at 'Will' and catches 'Will's eye, and in that moment something new is born; a connection happens, a light fires up, a moment of poignant clarity occurs, something is recognised.

'Will' catches her breath; she flushes and almost drops her eyes down; she hardly dares to hope. Her pointless life hovers around her as she struggles to hold the moment. She sits very still... and waits.

'I' looks away, of course.

For in that moment a truth is seen, a truth that endangers everything she knows, because if that truth is allowed, if 'I' lingers a moment longer, her world will turn upside down and everything will change.

Too much for 'I' just now. But for a fraction of a fraction of a second the world stilled and opened, and light flooded 'I's eyes, and really, yes, things have changed ... such a moment cannot be forgotten.

A question arises in 'I's confused mind: "what is that sitting over there... that silent wretched looking thing, so quiet and still? Is that me, or some nasty demon waiting to jump out at me? I think I have seen her before in the shadows of my mind, but always took her to be a mischief maker just out to cause me more trouble. But something happened when I caught her eye; a lightness and colour I haven't seen before, a spark of fire, a note of pearl blue. It seemed like magic; an intensity that frightened me... I had to look away ... and yet?... and yet?... and yet?..."

And yet... what?

Such a moment cannot be forgotten ... but it can be ignored.

This story has two endings:

Ending 1:

'I' dares...

to look again.

....

Ending 2:

'I' dares not... and hope fades into pointless and repetitive age; 'Will' gets used to being ignored and retires into hopeless oblivion, resigned to ill-use and loneliness, and 'Want', the child of 'Will', is never born.

———— ❧ ————

You do not fight with your mother ...

You do not fight *with* your mother ...

You fight with yourself, *for your mother's love.*

Intention: "I exist."

In the process:

'Exist' to the enquiring person: "I thought I was protecting myself from our mother, but I realise I am protecting myself from you."

Our survival from the traumas of not being wanted and not being loved leave us with a legacy of inner conflict, a fight for survival against the wishes of the mother, and a constant underlying fight for the love of our unloving mother.

But in this last, we end up fighting with ourselves for the love of our mother, because the reality is, we were not loved as a child, and yet we cannot accept this, and so we fight with ourselves for this idea that we can get her to love us. The conflict is within us.

Your body hears what is important to hear ...

Note-taking and other distractions.*

We think we have to capture everything, to remember everything in our process, and sometimes people write notes even while in the middle of their enquiry process.

However, once something is heard and felt in the body, it can never go. Your body is an organ of resonance, and remembers and registers everything, the trauma, the need to adjust for survival, and responds to and knows what is true, and what is false, and relaxes when things are right.

Whether you can put it into words or not is irrelevant. The information is there, it's been said and your body has responded, and that changes everything.

In fact, I would go so far as to say that in the process of taking something that has been said, and writing it down, we actually lose the reality of the thing said; we interrupt the physical resonance with what is said as we use our mind to construct it into words, into a sentence we can write down. We uphold the split between body and mind.

When you turn to write notes, you avoid the opportunity of real connection, you distract yourself with your notes away from the reality of the opportunity to come into contact and become truly who you are.

Who can feel the depth of their true feelings and write notes at the same time?

* Of course, this is when the process is being done online. It isn't possible to write notes when we are doing a process in person.

————— ∽ —————

Your heart is inside you ... beating

Intention: "I want my heart"

Understanding intentions is an important part of the IoPT facilitator's job. At the beginning of a process, we cannot say we understand the intention. To do so puts the facilitator in a position of expectation, and if we have expectations that we hold onto we are in danger of influencing the process, and we are lost as to the actual underlying meaning of the intention. As IoPT facilitators, we are here to learn what each intention actually means.

It is not unusual for the novice facilitator to make a snap decision about the intention from the beginning, because sitting in the place of not knowing is uncomfortable and to an extent re-stimulates our experience of helplessness, and that is our trauma re-triggered. This 'snap decision' more often than not takes the intention to mean what it seems to mean, but if we do that we fail. The point of the enquiry process is exactly that: for the facilitator, it is an enquiry to understand the less obvious, underlying specific meaning of the intention.

In addition, when we arrive at the end of the process, ideally the IoPT facilitator will understand the underlying meaning of the intention.

To think about an intention such as this, for example, involves understanding that a heart is a physical organ that functions to keep us alive. It beats and moves oxygen and blood around the body. So ,we could say "you already have your heart, otherwise you would be dead!"

Then we can think that the heart is a way of talking about love, and think about the intention as "I want love" or "I want my love". In such a configuration we may come to think that the word 'heart' actually may represent the mother as in "I want my mother".

This of course was the underlying issue: I cannot have my 'heart' if I am still longing for my mother ... I have given my heart to her.

In the end of the process we are back to the basic IoPT notion of the Trauma of Love, the lack of love of the mother for the child. This was captured in the phrase from one of the representatives:

"My mother stole my heart".

In this intention the word 'heart' is a concept, an idea. Your real heart is in your body, beating.

Your survival strategies are not the enemy

If you see your survival strategies as the enemy, you end up fighting windmills; you fight yourself, and you make these strategies that kept you alive, and in some cases still keep you alive, your foe.

They are not your enemy; the perpetrator was your enemy, at the very beginning of your life, and you developed survival strategies to manage and protect you from the trauma inflicted upon you by this perpetrator.

How much easier is it to overeat or take drugs than to face the reality of your trauma? How much easier is it to sit glued to your computer playing games or go shopping and spend money that you may not have, than confront the fact that you still long for the love you did not get? Easier to fail in your endeavours and succumb to depression than see that under it all, you were not wanted and you were not loved by the one person you needed to want you and love you. These are your survival strategies, your defence against your trauma, against such pain.

Even now, in the present, your trauma survival strategies protect you from what you cannot bear to know and feel in this moment. They moderate in each moment what you can tolerate and what you cannot.

Yes, they also limit your life, trip you up and perhaps even force you to turn on yourself and hurt and harm yourself ... and that is the point of taking yourself and your trauma, *and* your survival strategies seriously.

Your survival strategies call you to your trauma. They are the symptoms of trauma, and by the pain and suffering they cause you they summon you to take yourself and your trauma seriously. And when you do not need them anymore, they will simply disappear.

Ending ...

So, here we are at the end ... and the beginning of whatever comes next.

I hope you have enjoyed this book, and that it offers you something useful in your personal journey and your journey as an IoPT practitioner, if that applies to you. It has certainly been helpful to me to articulate many, at times, random thoughts and ideas that all have at their base perceptions about life and my work from an IoPT perspective. And it has been enjoyable to write about these ideas and share them with you.

IoPT is a psychology, extending into a philosophy that can help and guide us towards the healing of trauma, recognising that you were just a child, looking for love, and then moving towards living a good life.

I wish you a good life!

Vivian

References

Bentsen, A. (2017). Blog post: Contact Forms, Confluence and Introjection, on website Emerge Counselling and Consulting: https://www.emergecounseling.com/single-post/2017/05/29/contact-forms-confluence-introjection.

Broughton, V. (2012). Thinking About Ethics, unpublished paper.

Broughton, V. (2010) *In the Presence of Many: Reflections on Constellations Emphasising the Individual Context,* Green Balloon Publishing, UK.

Broughton, V. (2013). *The Heart of Things: Understanding trauma.* Green Balloon Publishing, UK.

Broughton, V. (2017). *Becoming your True Self: A handbook for the journey from trauma to healthy autonomy.* Green Balloon Publishing, UK.

Broughton, V. (2021). *Trauma and Identity: IoPT theory and practice.* Green Balloon Publishing, UK.

Crews, F. (2017). *Freud: The making of an illusion.* Profile Books, USA.

Freud, S. (1962). The Aetiology of Hysteria (1896) in *The Complete Psychological Works of Sigmund Freud Standard Edition Volume 3* (2001), translated by J Strachey. Hogarth Press, UK.

Freud, S. (1922). Beyond the Pleasure Principle, in *Sigmund Freud: Beyond the Pleasure Principle and Other Writings* (2003). Penguin, USA.

Grossman, D. (2009). *On Killing: The psychological cost of learning to kill in war and society.* E-Rights/E-Read, USA.

Herman, J.L. (1992). *Trauma and Recovery: The aftermath of violence - from domestic abuse to political terror.* Basic Books, USA.

Holmes, J. (1993). *John Bowlby & Attachment Theory.* Routledge, UK.

Kardiner, A., & **Spiegel,** H. (1947, Republished 2013). *War Stress and Neurotic Illness.* Isha Books, USA.

Makesy, C. (2022). *The Boy, the Mole, the Fox and the Horse.* Ebury Press, UK.

Marche, S. (2022). *The Next Civil War: Dispatches from the American Future.* Avid Reader Press, Simon Schuster, USA.

Masson, J. (1992). *The Assault on Truth: Freud and child sex abuse.* Harper Collins, USA.

McGilchrist, I. (2010). *The Master and his Emissary: The divided brain and the making of the western world.* Yale University Press, USA.

Miller, A. (1987). *For Your Own Good: The roots of violence in child-rearing.* Virago Press, London.

Ruppert, F. (2011). *Splits in the Soul: Integrating traumatic experiences.* English translation edited by V. Broughton. Green Balloon Publishing, UK.

Ruppert, F. (2019). *Who Am I in a Traumatised and Traumatising Society?* English translation edited by V. Broughton. Green Balloon Publishing, UK.

Ruppert, F. (2020). *Love, Lust and Trauma: The journey towards a healthy sexual identity.* English translation edited by V. Broughton. Published by Green Balloon Publishing, UK.

Ruppert, F. (2021). *I want to Live, Love and Be Loved.* Tredition GmbH, Germany.

Schore, A. N. (2012). *The Science of the Art of Psychotherapy.* Norton & Company, New York and London.

Stern, D.N. (1985). *The Interpersonal World of the Infant: A view from psychoanalysis and developmental psychology.* Routledge, USA.

Van der Kolk, B. A. (2007a). The History of Trauma in Psychiatry, in *Handbook of PTSD: Science and practice.* Edited by Friedman, M.J., Keane, T.M., Resick, P.A. Guildford Press, USA.

Whitfield, C.L. (1995). *Memory and Abuse: Remembering and healing the effects of trauma.* Health Communications Inc, USA.

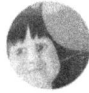

Green Balloon Publishing

By Franz Ruppert:

Trauma, Bonding & Family Constellations: *Understanding and healing injuries of the soul* (2008)

Splits in the Soul: *Integrating traumatic experiences* (2011)

Symbiosis & Autonomy: *Symbiotic trauma and love beyond entanglement* (2012)

Trauma, Fear and Love: *How the Constellation of the Intention supports healthy autonomy* (2014)

Early Trauma: *Pregnancy, birth and first years of life* (2016)

My Body, My Trauma, My I: *Setting up intentions, exiting our traumabiography* (2018)

Who Am I in a Traumatised and Traumatising Society? (2019)

Love Lust & Trauma: *The journey towards a healthy sexual identity* (2020)

By Vivian Broughton:

In the Presence of Many: *Reflections on constellations emphasising the individual context* (2010)

The Heart of Things: *Understanding trauma – working with constellations* (2013)

becoming your true self: *a handbook for the journey from trauma to healthy autonomy* (2014)

Trauma & Identity: *IOPT theory & practice* (2021)

www.greenballoonbooks.co.uk
info@greenballoonbooks.co.uk